D1245460

easy tai ji

any age • any place • any time

Robert Parry

Illustrated by
Juliet Percival

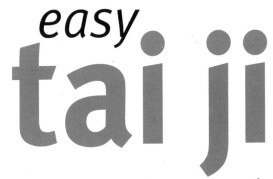

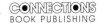
CONNECTIONS
BOOK PUBLISHING

A CONNECTIONS EDITION
This edition published in Great Britain in 2008 by
Connections Book Publishing Limited
St Chad's House, 148 King's Cross Road
London WC1X 9DH
www.connections-publishing.com

British Library Cataloguing-in-Publication data available on request.

ISBN 978-1-85906-269-2

1 3 5 7 9 10 8 6 4 2

The text in *Easy Tai Ji* is from *The Tai Chi Manual* by Robert Parry, published by Piatkus (1997). The illustrations are based on photographs by Laura Knox.

Phototypeset in Meta using QuarkXPress on Apple Macintosh
Printed in China

Contents

Introduction

Tai ji is fast becoming one of the most popular forms of fitness training in the world today – but it is not just about fitness. Tai ji is also a special way of looking at life – a path of inspiration and a guide towards relaxation and health. Daily practice will not only increase your sense of well-being and help you to deal with the stresses of modern living, but will also release enormous amounts of creativity and help you to stay bright, optimistic and alert from youth right through to old age.

This may sound miraculous, but it's true! It's why tai ji has stood the test of time, and why today – in homes and gardens, parks and recreation centres all over the world – people from all walks of life, all ages and all levels of fitness continue to practise its slow, graceful movements with as much enthusiasm and fondness as they have throughout so much of recorded history.

WHAT IS TAI JI?

Although it might appear to be tailor-made for dealing with the modern world and its relentless pressures, tai ji has in fact been around for a considerable length of time. With its origins rooted in ancient China, this integrated exercise system for body, mind and spirit has elements dating back as far as 3000 BCE. The translation of 'tai' is 'big' or 'great', while 'ji' is 'ultimate' or 'pure'. Tai ji, therefore, is all about experiencing something great and special through movement – namely the 'qi' (pronounced 'chi') that is the ultimate energy which powers the universe, from the greatest star right down to the smallest of microscopic creatures.

This book shows you how to discover and experience this kind of energy for yourself. If practised daily, tai ji will help you to maintain health and well-being, to stay relaxed and even to ward off some of the ravages of time. There is no expensive equipment to buy, no special clothing required. You already have everything you need – the natural qi of the body, available to you at all times; it's just a question of learning how to use it. Become part of it, and you will be linking into an amazing source of energy and liberation. In fact, just by opening this book you've taken the first step on a unique journey of self-discovery that could last for the rest of your life.

Tai ji is, of course, a martial art – and a very effective one, too! The martial arts flourished in China during the Middle Ages, when people blended the familiar techniques of punching, kicking and striking with the long and venerable tradition of therapeutic exercise that had developed over the centuries. Medical knowledge of the energy structure of the human body was then added, and the result was the birth of what became known as 'tai ji quan' (or 'tai chi chuan'). Many of tai ji's greatest living exponents are, in fact, martial artists of a very high calibre indeed.

In recent times, however, there has been a huge resurgence of interest in the original principles of energy flow which underlie tai ji, and this has led many people, drawn by tai ji's inherent grace and beauty, to explore once again its healing and inspirational qualities. It is this very factor that is the motivation behind this book.

THE SHORT YANG FORM

This book deals in depth with one of the most popular and easy-to-learn styles of tai ji – the short yang form, named after its founder Yang Lu Chuan. This is a simplified version of one of the more traditional forms that developed in China during the eighteenth and nineteenth centuries. The short form was in fact created in the earlier half of the twentieth century by Master Cheng Man-ch'ing (1900–1975) – a truly remarkable man who was not only a superb exponent of tai ji, but also a professor of literature, an expert in the use of Chinese herbs, a poet, a calligrapher and a painter. His condensed version of the yang style of tai ji, developed to suit his own busy schedule, has been his greatest gift to the world.

Many of the movements, based on the observation of animals, are of considerable antiquity (for example, *crane spreads its wings*). There are cave paintings depicting similar exercises dating from 200 BCE, while the legendary Yellow Emperor of China is said to have practised exercises for health based on the movements of animals as far back as 2700 BCE. Other movements have less elaborate, more self-explanatory names, attributed over the centuries through their use between teacher and pupil (for example, *turn and cross hands*).

HOW TO USE THIS BOOK

Whether you learn tai ji in a class situation from a teacher, or whether you choose to learn the basics from a book first and then take it further with personal tuition at a later date, the method of learning is usually the same, and hasn't altered much throughout the ages. Students begin by assimilating each of the basic individual movements, one at a time, and then, once familiar with them, put them all together to create the beautiful flowing sequence that most of us recognize as typical of tai ji. This book continues in that tradition – but contains some exciting new departures.

Here, the sequence itself is divided into seven clearly defined segments, (traditionally it is taught only in two parts). This results in a clear, step-by-step approach, with easy 'bite-sized' chunks of the form that can be absorbed before going on to the next stage. You can practise as little or as often as suits you. Each lesson focuses on different aspects of movement, beginning with balance and mastering basic stances, through to moving backwards and sideways, twisting and turning, and finally integrating all the skills you have learnt to achieve a combination of agility, strength and grace.

Each stance is also accompanied by a detailed foot diagram, indicating the required position, orientation and weight distribution for that stance, so that you know exactly where – and how – to step. Together with the clear, concise instructions, all this ensures that the movements are easy to follow, and creates a highly user-friendly book containing everything you need to get started on your tai ji journey.

Once you have worked your way through all the stages, and are familiar with the whole sequence, you may find that you no longer need to refer back to the book for step-by-step instruction. The wall chart shown on the inside of the book jacket provides a handy reference aid to the entire short yang form, and is a great memory-jogger for when you don't want to stop to consult the book mid-sequence. The chart is colour-coded to match the book, so that you can easily turn to the relevant lesson and step number, if you need to refer to the full instructions at any stage.

HOW LONG DOES IT TAKE TO LEARN?

Nature does not reveal her secrets lightly; tai ji, being rooted so deeply in the natural world, requires a reasonable commitment of time and energy. Ideally, you'll need to practise a little every day to achieve results. Once learnt, however, the whole sequence takes only about 8 minutes to perform, which, together with a brief warm-up session, will bring your commitment to around just 10 minutes daily. This 10 minutes will never be wasted. It will repay you over and over again in terms of health and well-being.

Although you will start to feel the benefits of practising tai ji fairly early on, most people who study the short yang form need about six months to a year to learn it all the way through. Give yourself time to assimilate the movements properly; remember that with each lesson you will be developing your skills and encountering new types of movement, and you'll find it easier if you are completely comfortable with the movements in one section before you go on to the next.

And the learning process doesn't stop once you've learnt the form – this is the beauty and the fascination of tai ji. There is no limit to how far it can take you, so that as each hill is climbed, another even more interesting one comes into view. That's tai ji. Now give it a try!

getting started

Before you learn the movements of the form, you need to be
familiar with the basic principles of tai ji practice – standard foot
and hand positions, and things you should and shouldn't do.
This section introduces typical tai ji stances, and also includes
exercises for that all-important warm-up, to loosen up your joints
and warm your muscles before you begin your tai ji. You can
repeat the exercises as many times as desired. Always wear
loose, comfortable clothing and footwear that won't
slide about too much.

Warming up

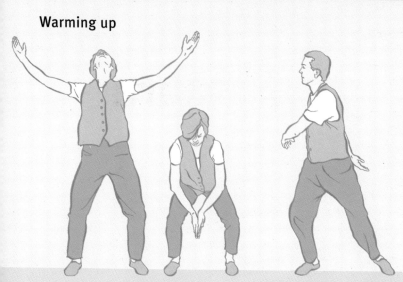

COMPLETE STRETCH With your knees slightly bent, spread your arms wide and lean slightly backwards as you breathe in (*above left*), then straighten up, bring your hands together, palms up initially, then back-to-back as you breathe out and squat down (*above centre*). As you move, swoop your hands (still back-to-back) down between your knees and then part them as you straighten your back again and breathe in. Open your arms wide once more as you come up, and then carry on by repeating the same movement a few more times.

TWISTING With your feet and knees wide apart, gently twist your body from side to side, allowing your arms to relax and swing around as you turn. The movements should come from the centre of the body, not from the shoulders or arms. Relax your shoulders, and let your arms go very loose, so that they wind around your body as you turn. Increase the size of the rotation by raising the opposite heel each time (simply transfer your weight as you twist). All the while, make sure you keep your knees apart, rather like sitting on a horse.

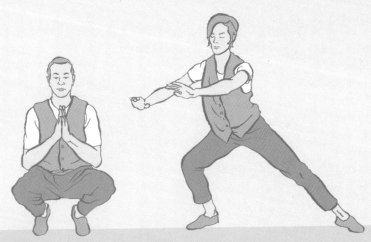

SQUATTING Bring your palms together and then, keeping the movement as slow as you can, squat down – not too far at first – raising your heels and bending your knees as you go. Don't worry if you feel stiff to begin with; you will find that you're gradually able to increase the depth to which you can squat. You may also hear cracking from your knees – that's OK! It simply means that you are clearing out congested energy from the joints. (If you are especially stiff, you may find it easier to hold onto a chair with one hand as you squat down.)

TURNING THE WHEEL Squat down on one side only, stretching the other leg straight as you go. Imagine that your hands are holding an imaginary wheel as you squat down, with your palms held out, relaxed and wide – not tense – and with lots of space between your arms and your body. Try to feel the work along your inside leg. Repeat this movement as desired. Then pause, bring your weight into your other foot, and repeat the exercise the same number of times on the other side.

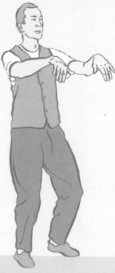

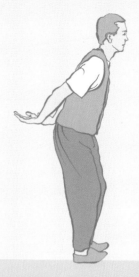

ROTATING HANDS AND FEET Holding your hands out in front of you, with your fingers loose and pointing down, slowly rotate your hands (in opposite directions) from the wrist joint, keeping the rotational movements large but your forearms still. Then pause, and continue the rotations in the reverse direction. To finish, shake your hands vigorously to really loosen them up.

For the feet, raise each foot in turn and slowly rotate it from the ankle joint in both directions, again keeping the movements large but the knee still. Gently shake out each foot after rotating it, to finish.

ROCKING ON HEELS AND TOES With a good bend to the knees, swing your arms and allow your body to rock very gently back and forth by raising both heels as you rock forward, and raising the toes of both feet as you rock backward. Again, the movement should come from the centre of the body, so keep those shoulders relaxed! Rotate the hands during each swing, so that the palms are always turned up at the finish, front and back, providing extra rotations for those all-important wrist joints.

Basic stances and hand work

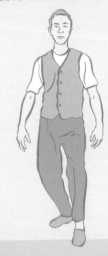

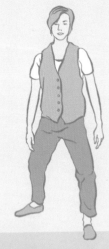

NARROW STANCES A narrow stance means that most of your weight (90 per cent) is in your rear leg, with either the toes of the front foot (a narrow toe stance) or the heel of the front foot (a narrow heel stance) in light contact with the ground ahead of you. In both cases the front foot is roughly in line with the edge of the back heel.

THE WIDE 70/30 STANCE '70/30' refers to the ratio of weight between the feet, with roughly 70 per cent in one leg and 30 in the other. The greater part of your weight can be either forward, in the front leg, or back, in the rear leg. The term 'wide' means the width across your shoulders from tip to tip. In 70/30 stances, you always strive to keep this amount of space between your feet, regardless of any length between the front and the back foot (so, when seen from the front, the feet should always be shoulder-width apart). It's rather like standing on (narrow!) railway lines.

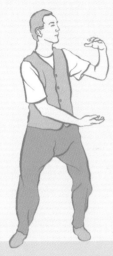

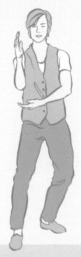

HOLDING THE BALL When learning many of the tai ji movements, it's often helpful to visualize a ball being held in various ways between your hands. This ensures a good energy connection between the palms, which, in time, you will begin to feel. Of course, the ball itself doesn't always have to be strictly spherical in shape; sometimes it becomes stretched or compressed, while at others small or large. This principle of communication between the hands and arms continues throughout almost the entire form.

CUPPING THE ELBOW This is a configuration that appears quite often in various guises throughout the tai ji form. Here, you do not literally cup or support the elbow in any physical sense; rather, the palm is a good distance from the elbow itself, and roughly in line with the vital centre of your body situated in your abdomen (in China this is known as the *Dan Tien* and in Japan as the *Hara – see also page 15*). The fingers of the lower hand should be relaxed, while the top hand can be either flat in shape, or gently curved over.

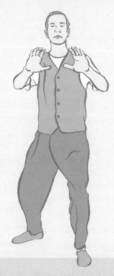
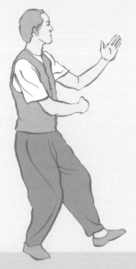

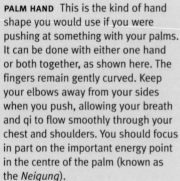

PALM HAND This is the kind of hand shape you would use if you were pushing at something with your palms. It can be done with either one hand or both together, as shown here. The fingers remain gently curved. Keep your elbows away from your sides when you push, allowing your breath and qi to flow smoothly through your chest and shoulders. You should focus in part on the important energy point in the centre of the palm (known as the *Neigung*).

FLAT HAND Here, the fingers straighten out to give a flattened appearance. It is not often encountered in the form, but when it is, it must not become a source of tension. Although the fingers are fairly straight compared to most tai ji movements, they should not become rigid and stiff. This allows the qi to keep flowing, from the shoulders right through to the fingertips.

Dos and don'ts

KEEP THE SPINE UPRIGHT
Traditionally, when you learn tai ji, you are told to imagine a point of suspension situated on the crown of the head. From this, a golden thread goes up to the heavens, so that you move as if suspended, always vertical. Alternatively, think of the base of the spine as a bob on the end of a plumb line. No matter whether the plumb line moves forward or back, the string always remains upright.

NEVER TIGHTLY LOCK THE ELBOWS OR KNEES This goes for all the joints in the body. Think of water in a hosepipe: when the pipe has a twist or bend in it, the water ceases to flow smoothly, or may stop altogether. The same applies to the qi in the body. Maintaining relaxed and flexible limbs, without tension, enables blood and bodily fluids to flow easily and without obstruction.

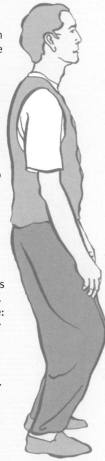

MOVE FROM THE CENTRE Our vital energy centre is situated in the abdomen – a point just below the navel called the *Dan Tien*. In tai ji, all of the turns, steps and rotations should be directed from here – like a searchlight guiding the movements of the limbs. Try to direct your breathing down into this area: imagine the essence of the breath sinking to the *Dan Tien*, a constant focus of attention. Retain this quality of self-awareness in your practice.

MAINTAIN A LOW CENTRE OF GRAVITY When you do your tai ji, always allow your weight to sink down. A slight bend to the knees helps to create the typical tai ji appearance, which is somewhat low-slung and stealth-like. This quality should be cultivated during all of your work, so that the movements flow one into the other without bobbing up or down.

DROP THE SHOULDERS

This isn't always easy to do for those who suffer from stress, because the shoulders tend to collect tension very easily – and then surrender it only very grudgingly, despite our best efforts! However, tai ji provides an excellent opportunity to correct bad habits and to dispel areas of accustomed tension. Therefore, as your arms move – and especially as they rise – try not to let your shoulders rise up with them. If you do allow your shoulders to rise, you will end up in a hunched, rigid posture, rather than the relaxed, open posture that you're aiming for.

KEEP SPACE BETWEEN YOUR ARMS AND YOUR BODY

In tai ji, there should always be a generous amount of space under the arms, leaving the armpits with an open feeling. Also, the elbows should not come into contact with the sides at any time. All this frees off the chest and rib-cage; it allows you to breathe more easily and encourages the energy to flow more smoothly along the arms. Don't overdo this, though – we're not seeking the 'gorilla' look here! You simply need to adopt a posture of openness and relaxation.

STEP FORWARD HEEL FIRST

Always step forward making contact with the heel first, and not the toes. Conversely, when you step back your toes should make contact first. This ensures a smooth action and is, in fact, the way the legs like to unbend naturally, with the least number of adjustments among the joints. Also, after any step forward always be ready to adjust the back foot to a comfortable position by pivoting a little on the back heel; if your heel will not turn, and you can only pivot on the ball of your foot, there is usually one simple explanation: you have stepped too narrow.

FRONT KNEE OVER TOES

In wide stances, when you bring your weight forward, make sure the knee doesn't extend beyond the toes on the front foot. This would only create instability in your stance. Rather, always try to keep the knee and toes in alignment; for most of us, because of the line-of-sight effect, the toes should just disappear beneath the knee as you look down.

KEEP THE KNEE ABOVE THE FRONT FOOT

In wide stances, make sure that your knee remains above what is called the 'substantial' foot – the one carrying the weight – and isn't turned or twisted inwards. Rather, always try to keep your thigh, knee, shin and foot in line; weakness of the energies that flow along the inside of the leg can be responsible for any difficulty in achieving this position. Try to be aware of this and correct it by spiralling the knee back over the foot.

DON'T STAND TOO NARROW

Make sure your narrow stances aren't too narrow. As a rule, the front foot should always be roughly in a line with the edge of the back heel, and not too close to it in terms of length, either. Try to be generous with this type of stance, and make sure that the thigh, knee, shin and foot are all aligned, so that your foot doesn't protrude out to the side in a twisted fashion. Try not to introduce any unnecessary tension by raising the heels or toes too much.

TROUBLESHOOTING

You need to maintain this proper alignment during your tai ji practice, in order for the vital energy to flow unimpeded through the entire body. In times of doubt, or whenever you suspect your tai ji isn't flowing smoothly, refer back to this section to check that you're not doing something fundamentally wrong to upset your equilibrium.

---

the short yang form

You are now going to begin learning the individual movements which, when added together, ultimately transform themselves into the elegant, flowing sequence known as the short yang form. The form has a beginning and an end, and whenever it is performed the movements are always repeated in the same order. It's useful to compare this to a graceful slow-motion dance, or to a piece of music that always continues from its beginning to its inevitable conclusion with a constant and even tempo throughout.

Rhythm and tempo are the keys to fluent tai ji technique. The rhythm is one we are all very familiar with: the rhythm of the breath. When we're very relaxed and calm, our breathing becomes long and regularly spaced; conversely, when we're excited or angry, our breathing becomes rapid and irregular. In tai ji we cultivate regular breathing coupled with slow, carefully measured movements, so that, in time, we become more internally balanced and harmonized with the natural world.

Following the form

Once you're familiar with the basic stances and principles, you are ready to begin learning the form itself. All the movements are clearly illustrated, showing both the yin phase (the 'yielding' aspect which accompanies the in-breath) and the yang phase (the 'thrust' of the movement which accompanies the out-breath). If you pay close attention to the positions shown and read the instructions carefully, you'll find it easy to follow the movements yourself. Remember: be patient. Learn each section thoroughly before going on to the next, and think in terms of months rather than weeks for learning the form all the way through.

Although the entire sequence should take around 8 minutes to perform, it can be done more slowly if you wish. Beginners tend to be a little faster than the more advanced students, although Master Cheng himself used to do it in 5 minutes or less! The main thing is to feel relaxed with what you are doing, and bear in mind that extreme slowness can introduce more tension than it removes. Find your own pace, and let this take you wherever you need to go.

FOOT POSITIONS
The foot diagrams show the corresponding position, orientation and weight distribution for each stance. The foot bearing the higher percentage of weight is labelled in each case, and the shaded area indicates the part of the foot in contact with the ground.

Against these diagrams you will find the cardinal directions of north, south, east and west (except on the diagrams that accompany stances involved in moving from one direction to another). These are traditionally used by tai ji teachers to help students find the correct orientation. Here, they are given as a guide only, to help with the learning process; in practice, this is preferable to continually referring to left and right, which can become confusing. You don't literally have to face these directions. When dotted lines are shown, these indicate a change of position – that a step has taken place; the dots show the location of the previous stance.

BREATHING

Each movement is accompanied by instructions for breathing. Don't force yourself to follow these if you feel at all uncomfortable. Begin by finding your own rhythm of inhalation and exhalation; you will gradually begin to tune in to the breathing patterns given. Remember that in tai ji the learning process should always be one of discovery and fun – so relax and enjoy it!

A DEEPER LEVEL

Tai ji has a strong mental and even spiritual aspect. It's not essential for you to explore these areas in order to obtain the wonderful benefits that tai ji can bring in terms of physical health and relaxation, but they will help you find a deeper satisfaction and enjoyment in what you are doing.

It all comes down to understanding the original concept of the universal 'Tai Ji' – the supreme ultimate – often depicted as a circle divided by a graceful curve (the 'Tai Ji Tu', familiar to most of us as the yin/yang symbol), suggesting movement and change. 'Change' is the key word. The light half of the circle is yang, the dark half yin; these two forces, the positive and negative forces of nature, balance and complement each other perfectly in a state of continual harmony. Each one nourishes and supports the other in a perpetual rhythm of change.

Translated into physical movement, this gives us the tai ji form, which alternates constantly between negative and positive forces, accompanied by the in-breath (yin) and the out-breath (yang), so that the changes take place at a very deep level. Your tai ji is a reflection and celebration of nature, of great universal forces and rhythms with which we can work in harmony to benefit ourselves, not only physically but mentally and emotionally as well.

the early moves

The early movements of the form are all about developing balance and becoming aware of your own personal space. Wide 70/30 stances feature heavily throughout this section, so always keep in mind those ' railway lines' : your feet should be shoulder-width apart when you step, regardless of any length between one foot and the other.

1 Preparation

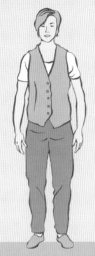

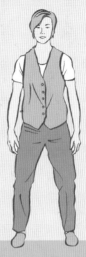

BREATHE IN

1 Face south to begin, your back straight and shoulders relaxed.

2 Make sure you're not leaning forwards or backwards, or to one side. Your hips should be level and your arms hanging loosely by your sides, rather than pressed close to your body. Keep your bottom tucked in, and your neck straight by tucking in your chin a little.

3 Slowly, empty your weight from your left side and allow your left foot to lift and then slide out to the left.

BREATHE OUT

1 Set your left foot down, shoulder-width from your right with your toes pointing south, then adjust your right toes to also point south, just before allowing your weight to settle evenly into both feet.

2 Relax and imagine your weight sinking down. Keep your back straight, not leaning forward, not leaning back.

3 Think of the plumb line (*see page 15*), and allow your spine to hang perfectly vertically, as if it were suspended from above.

❷ Opening

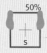

50%

S

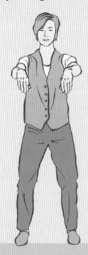

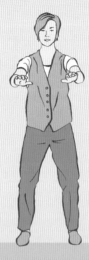

50%

S

BREATHE IN

1 With your wrists and fingers loose, raise your forearms, as if floating in water, until they become roughly parallel to the ground. Don't let your shoulders rise up as well – this will only introduce tension.

2 Be aware of how even these fairly simple movements might affect other parts of the body; the loose wrists, for example, inform your body straight away that you intend to relax your arms. All this makes a difference to the way you feel about the movements.

BREATHE OUT

1 Slowly straighten your fingers. Imagine the energy coming from between your shoulders to straighten your fingers as you exhale.

2 As you do this, make sure your palms don't lift or appear to push forward. It's sometimes more helpful to think of the wrists dropping rather than the fingers rising. Dropping the wrists is a 'letting go' kind of movement, which is preferable to the more tensile operation involved in raising the fingers.

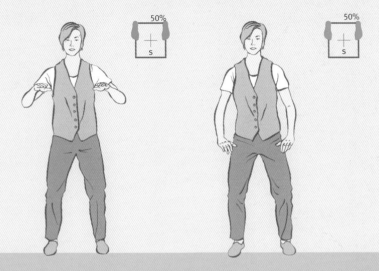

BREATHE IN

1 Draw your elbows back a little – not too far, otherwise the area behind, between your shoulder blades, could become tense.

2 Don't lean back as your elbows withdraw; only your arms should move. Make sure you keep space between your arms and sides. This allows the breath to flow easily in the chest.

3 Recognize your own personal space and make room for yourself! Don't forget that tai ji works on all levels: physical, mental and emotional.

BREATHE OUT

1 Lower your arms and sink down, letting your knees bend a little more and keeping your back straight. Don't lean.

2 Relax your shoulders, chest and arms, and imagine your weight sinking into the ground. Think of pushing a ball down through water as you do this, but remember: whenever you hear the word 'push' in tai ji it is always meant to be without muscular tension, with the arms remaining light at all times.

❸ Turn right

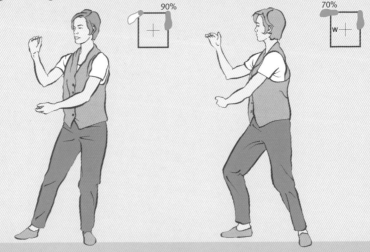

BREATHE IN

1 Empty the weight from your right side by sinking into your left foot.

2 Slowly pivot on your right heel to point your toes west. At the same time, raise your right forearm and begin to cup your right elbow with your left palm as your waist turns towards the right; your right hand should be loosely curved.

3 Remember the terminology here: in cupping the elbow (*see page 13*), the hand does not literally make contact with the elbow or support it in any physical sense.

BREATHE OUT

1 Bend your right knee to align with the tip of your foot. You might find that your left knee wants to bend a little too. Let it go. Relax!

2 Your head, hips and shoulders should now have turned towards the west, with your hands moving position slightly to hold an imaginary ball, the right hand curved over on top of the ball, and the left hand supporting it from underneath.

3 Meanwhile, direct your gaze outwards, just over your right hand, as if looking towards a far-off horizon.

④ Ward off

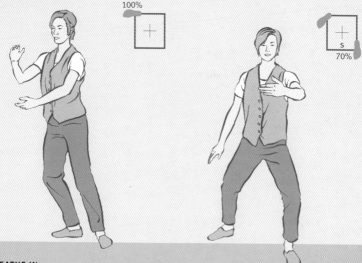

BREATHE IN

1 Prepare to step ahead, towards the south, by bringing all your weight into your right leg and drawing in your left toes just a little towards your right heel. This drawing in of the toes is a typical preparation for moving into a wide stance and helps to test your balance before stepping – which you will do on the out-breath, by extending your left leg out towards the south.

2 Turn the right palm forward just a little, ready to 'stroke' downwards.

BREATHE OUT

1 Step forward with your left foot and turn your waist towards the south, so that your centre is facing forward. This is the first of our 70/30 stances (*see page 12*), so you will need to place your foot outwards good and wide.

2 At the same time, raise your left arm, the forearm horizontal, palm facing in towards the chest, while dropping your right hand to the side.

3 Finally, pivot inwards a little on your right heel, to release any tension in the back knee.

5 Grasp the bird's tail

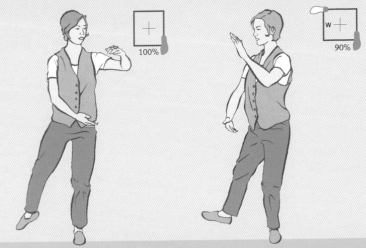

100%

w 90%

BREATHE IN

1 Begin by turning your waist slightly to the left and then pick up another imaginary ball, this time with the left hand on top.

2 Empty the weight from your right side and prepare to step by drawing your right toes in a little towards your left heel. It's worth noting that the image of the 'ball' here, as elsewhere, is just to get you started; these movements will soon feel natural on their own.

IN-BREATH FINISHES

1 Sink into your left leg, lift your right foot from the ground and, turning your waist clockwise, step around to the west, heel first.

2 As you do this, the ball goes with you, and the in-breath is completed; your heel should make contact with the ground just as the out-breath begins. Notice how the fingers of the left hand become more upright as the heel touches back down.

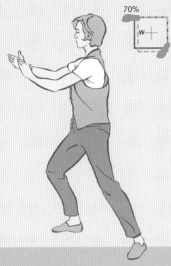

70%

BREATHE OUT

1 Bend your right knee to bring your weight forward and adjust your back heel to a comfortable position.

2 At the same time, close up the imaginary ball, until you finish with your right arm slanting upwards at a gentle angle and the fingers of your left hand pointing at the right palm.

3 Now imagine holding a bird in your right palm, while your left hand rests on the long tail feathers behind.

NOTE:

This is the first of a sequence of movements that occurs four times in total throughout the form – rather like the chorus in a piece of music. The movements are shown in detail here; you can refer back to this section if you find you need to refresh your memory when the chorus appears again later on in the form.

⑥ Rollback and press

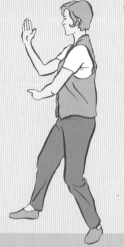

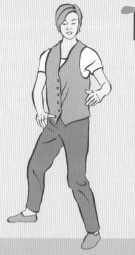
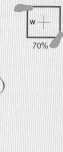

BREATHE IN

1 Begin by shifting your weight into the back leg. Rotate your hands slightly as you 'slide' your left hand down your right forearm at a distance, to cup your right elbow. The angle at the elbow becomes a little more acute as your right hand flattens out.

2 As you do this, turn your waist ever so slightly to the right. Make sure your left arm doesn't crowd in on your centre.

IN-BREATH FINISHES

1 Turn your waist anticlockwise and circle your left hand back behind you, while your right forearm folds down across your centre. Most of your weight is now in the back leg, and your left hand should be fairly relaxed in shape as compared to the right.

2 Try to cultivate a feeling of contact between the palms as you go through this manoeuvre, as if you can sense the energetic connection between the hands.

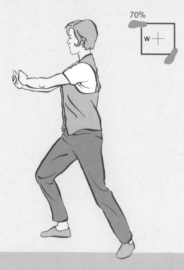

70%

BREATHE OUT

1 Rotate your palms to face each other, then bend your right knee and turn your waist back towards the west.

2 As you return your weight to your right side, allow your left palm to approach the right until the heels of the palms (the fleshy part at the base) make contact in front of your chest. Most of the hand energy is now concentrated in your left hand, to mirror the energy of the right leg.

⑦ Separate hands and push

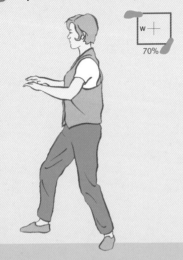

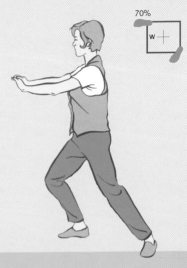

BREATHE IN

1 Rotate your hands so that your palms are facing downwards, then separate them outwards and back with a little swimming motion as you sit back once again into the rear leg, making sure you don't lock the front knee as you go.

2 Your hands should be relaxed, with your thumbs pointing towards the sides of the chest, as if you're about to tuck them into your braces (although don't overdo this!). As always, aim to create a relaxed appearance to the movement.

BREATHE OUT

1 Rotate your palms into a pushing position, then return your weight slowly forwards by bending your right knee.

2 Your hands should be covering the centre of your body, with your thumbs almost pointing towards each other; this helps to take the elbows away from the sides and enables the breath and the qi to flow comfortably in the chest.

3 Don't lean forward with the push; keep your back straight. The 'push' comes from the legs, not the arms.

8 Single whip

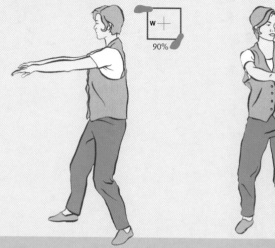
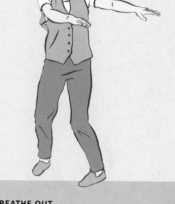

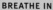

BREATHE IN

1 Sit back on the rear leg and allow your arms to straighten, though not so far as to lock the elbows. Your palms should be facing down.

2 Don't straighten your arms by 'diving' forward; all you need to do is keep your arms relaxed and in the same place that they were at the end of the push. As you sit back they will automatically straighten for you. Remember: tai ji is without effort.

BREATHE OUT

1 With the weight mostly in your left side, pivot very slowly on your right heel to turn your waist anticlockwise, allowing your arms to follow your centre as your waist turns around.

2 Don't go so far as to feel tense or 'wound up'; remember that all these movements should feel comfortable and agreeable.

3 Your feet should become slightly pigeon-toed as you turn, pointing in towards each other as if upon the sides of a triangle.

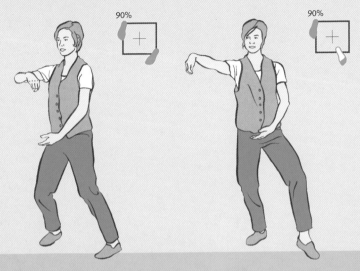

90%

90%

BREATHE IN

1 Your waist now reverses direction, rotating clockwise, while you draw your right hand across near to your right shoulder, forming a 'crane's beak' – a hook shape with the fingers and thumb lightly touching.

2 At the same time, swoop your left hand down, palm up, to settle near your right hip, as though to support a balloon from beneath, with the fingers of the right hand 'pinching' the neck of the balloon.

BREATHE OUT

1 With most of your weight now in your right side, raise your left heel and pivot on your toes, turning your waist anticlockwise as you do so.

2 As you do this, straighten your right arm (without locking the elbow) to project your crane's beak out towards the south-west, your gaze following your right hand as it goes. These movements encourage flexibility and relaxation in the wrists and elbows.

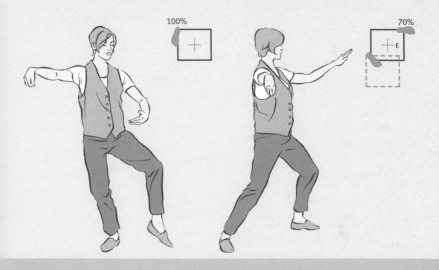

BREATHE IN

1 For the final stage, empty all the weight from your left side and prepare to step around with your left heel to the east.

2 Raise your left hand, palm facing in, looking at your palm as it rises to ensure the correct orientation of the arm. Let your elbow float.

3 Sink your weight into your right foot as you do this; then, when you feel balanced, draw your left toes in slightly towards your right heel, ready to step.

BREATHE OUT

1 Step around to the east with your left heel and bend your knee. As soon as the weight returns to your left side, pivot on your right heel to adjust your back foot to a comfortable position.

2 Meanwhile, rotate your left hand to point the fingers outwards. Your hand should be in line with the left side of the chest. The crane's beak remains a continual focus of energy throughout.

introducing narrow stances

In this section we meet with the narrow stances, in which most of the weight goes into the rear leg, with either the heel or the toes of the front foot in light contact with the ground. The focus here is on developing greater balance, both physically and mentally. Narrow stances are also an excellent preparation for the kicking sequences that occur later in the form.

9 Play guitar (right side)

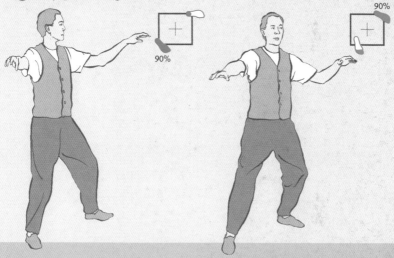

90%

90%

BREATHE IN

1 From the single whip (the point at which you finished the previous section), you now come to 'play guitar' – a narrow heel stance to the south. Don't let the name mislead you: the configuration of the arms is nothing like playing a guitar!

2 Begin by letting go of the crane's beak in your right hand, relax your arms, and turn your left toes inwards slightly by pivoting on your left heel. The left hand changes shape a little with this, just as you commence your inhalation.

IN-BREATH FINISHES

1 Shift your weight entirely into your left leg, keeping the knee bent and soft.

2 Rotate your waist a little towards the south (clockwise) and prepare for the final stage of the movement by raising your right heel, ready to draw your foot across in front of you. (Although at this point your right toes may still be in contact with the ground, they should be carrying hardly any weight.)

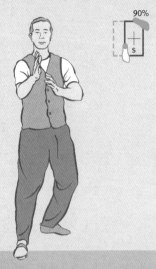

90%

BREATHE OUT

1 Lift up your toes and draw your right heel across to place it down in a narrow heel stance, hips and shoulders facing south.

2 At the same time, close your hands in towards each other, your right arm extended a little further in front of you than your left, until you finish with the palm of the left hand facing your right forearm.

3 Try to feel the energetic connection between your arms as they approach each other.

⑩ Pull and step with shoulder

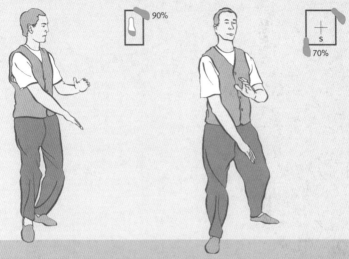

90%

70%

BREATHE IN

1 Lower your arms, rather like pulling a thick rope downwards with your hands, your left hand near your left hip and your right arm across your centre, almost vertical.

2 Simultaneously draw in your right toes, to place them just ahead of your left heel (this is about as close as the two feet ever come to each other in tai ji); your waist will turn slightly anticlockwise as you do this. Don't forget to leave some space between your arms and your body.

BREATHE OUT

1 Step wide with the right foot, transferring your weight, and rotate your waist a little more to your left as you go, so that your right shoulder appears to project forward – rather like someone barging down a door.

2 Keeping your right arm where it was in the previous stance, raise your left hand a little, roughly to the height of your lower ribs, palm slightly forward-facing but still maintaining a subtle energy connection with the right forearm. Your hips and shoulders should now be facing south-east.

⑪ Crane spreads its wings

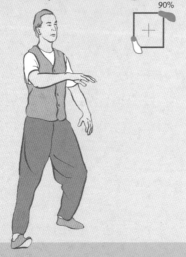

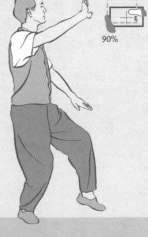

BREATHE IN

1 This movement is said to emulate the spreading and drying of a great bird's wings in the sunshine, and is one of the most beautiful and elegant of all tai ji stances. You are now preparing to move into a narrow toe stance towards the east.

2 Begin by pivoting a little on your right heel, to help direct your centre around to an east-facing position.

IN-BREATH FINISHES

1 As you form a narrow toe stance with your left foot, your arms become like great wings – broad, powerful and expansive. Drop your left hand, to hover above the left thigh, while raising your right hand to make an extravagant kind of salute, almost as if you were shielding your eyes from the sun.

2 Make sure you keep a little bit of energy in your left hand as well, in readiness to swap arms in the next step.

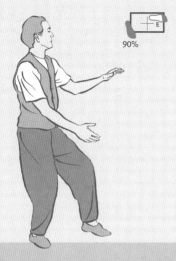

90%

BREATHE OUT

1 Keeping your feet still, change the wings by lowering your right arm and raising the left. Your arms should move in curves rather than in straight lines up or down – rather like turning a giant steering wheel.

2 Try to maintain the subtle energy connection between the palms as they pass each other, and feel the buoyant energy of the crane in your limbs.

⑫ Brush left knee and push

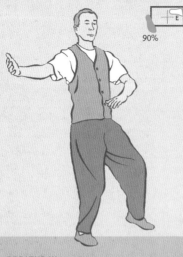

90%

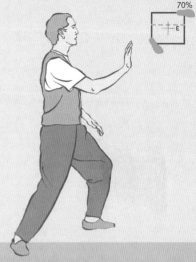

70%

BREATHE IN

1 Begin to turn your waist clockwise and allow the right 'wing' to circle back behind you, palm up at this stage – almost like holding an object in your right hand, ready to hurl.

2 Meanwhile, circle your left hand up and over towards your centre, in the process of making a small clockwise circle.

3 Keep your head and shoulders properly aligned with your hips. Focus your eyes on your right palm as it drifts backwards.

BREATHE OUT

1 Step wide with your left foot, and as you do this 'brush' across your left knee with your left palm, from right to left, turning your waist anticlockwise as you go.

2 Keep your left hand about 20 cm (8 in) away from your leg throughout this movement, then push out towards the east with your right hand, to finish in a wide 70/30 stance to the east. Your right palm should finish roughly in line with the centre of the chest, and not out to the side.

13 Play guitar (left side)

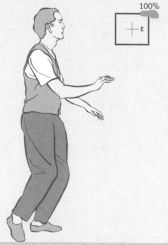

100%

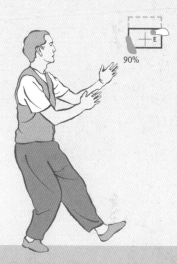

90%

BREATHE IN

1 Transferring all your weight into your left foot for a moment, allow your back foot to leave the ground and follow through, just a short way, rather like kicking a football with the inside of the foot. This is really a little side-step, to test your balance.

2 Now place your foot back down behind you again, in roughly the same place as it was before.

3 At the same time, relax your hands, your wrists dropping a little with the in-breath.

BREATHE OUT

1 Sitting back into the rear leg, draw your left heel across and place it down in a narrow stance ahead of your right foot.

2 As you do this, close your hands in on each other, this time with your left arm extended a little further than the right, with the palm of your right hand facing your left forearm.

3 Try to visualize your left palm in particular becoming energized, though keep it relaxed at the same time. Your hips and shoulders should still be facing east.

⑭ Brush left knee and push

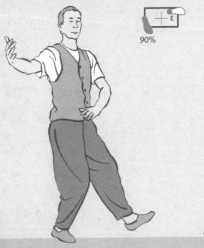

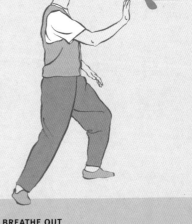

BREATHE IN

1 Relax your hands, turn your waist clockwise and circle your right palm back behind you.

2 As before (*see page 42*), from the corner of your eye watch your palm go back, keeping your head squared up with your shoulders as your waist turns. You will find that it really does help to visualize a light, flat object in your palm, as if ready to hurl. This will help you to achieve the correct orientation of the right hand more easily.

BREATHE OUT

1 Return your centre to the east once more by rotating your waist anticlockwise, and step out – good and wide – with the left foot.

2 Brush your left knee with your left palm as you go (remembering the distance between your palm and leg), and then push out east with your right palm as your left knee bends and your weight goes forward again.

3 Don't let the left hand 'flop' or drop away behind you once you have completed the brush knee.

15 Step forward, parry and punch

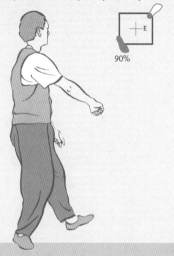

90%

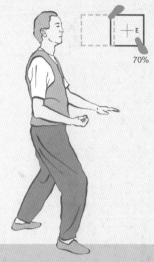

70%

BREATHE IN

1 As we go through this sequence we are going to count the movements of the feet – one, two and three – to make the learning process easier. Begin by forming a loose fist in your right hand – it should be rounded and clean in shape, but without tightness.

2 Lower your arms to the left side and, shifting your weight momentarily from your left foot, turn your left toes outwards by pivoting on the heel.

3 Put your left foot down flat on the ground and mentally count out the number one.

BREATHE OUT

1 Step forward with your right foot, planting it down with the toes pointing out, roughly south-east. Mentally count out the number two.

2 With this, 'throw' the fist in a graceful arc across your centre and round to your right hip, to finish with the knuckle side of the hand pointing downwards. Your left palm follows to settle in the centre, your arm almost horizontal at this stage.

3 Now bring your weight over into your right side by bending your right knee.

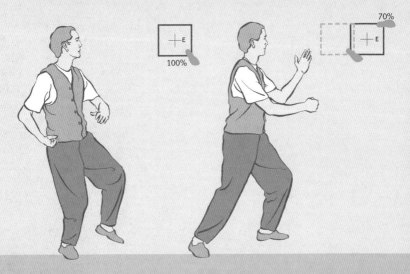

BREATHE IN

1 With your weight now in your right side, lift your left foot and prepare to step forward towards the east by drawing your toes in just a little towards your right heel.

2 Allow your waist to turn slightly in a clockwise direction, and draw back the fist in your right hand, knuckles still facing downward, ready to punch.

3 At the same time, begin to raise your left forearm, ready to parry – that is, to deflect an oncoming force away to the left-hand side.

BREATHE OUT

1 Step straight ahead with your left foot, and mentally count out the number three. This is your third and final step. As you do this, parry with the left forearm, sweeping out to the north from the centre.

2 As your left knee bends and your weight goes into it, project the fist forward to the east very slowly. Rotate it a quarter-turn as you go, to finish with the thumb side uppermost. Keep your arms relaxed.

3 Adjust your back heel to a comfortable position, if necessary.

16 Release arm and push

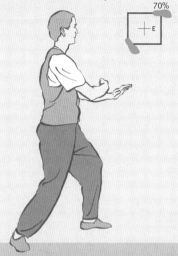

70%

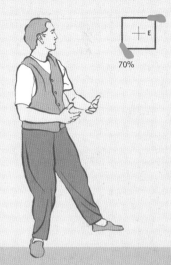

70%

BREATHE IN

1 With your right arm still extended, turn your waist a little to the left, and slide your left hand, palm down, beneath your right forearm.

2 Now let go of the fist in your right hand and turn both palms up. As you do this, reverse the turn in your waist, draw your right hand back across your left forearm and sit back into the rear leg.

3 Allow your left hand to follow the right, close to your centre.

IN-BREATH FINISHES

1 By the end of the inhalation your hands should be in the process of rotating into a palms-out position, ready to push forward, while your waist has turned slightly clockwise and the weight has transferred into the back leg.

2 Maintain an open aspect to the arms, with lots of space between your elbows and body.

3 Keep your spine straight, without leaning backwards, and don't lock the front knee.

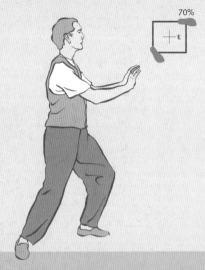

BREATHE OUT

1 Bend your left knee and bring your weight slowly forward again, as you push out to the east with your palms at about chest height.

2 Your thumbs should be pointing towards each other and your hands roughly covering the centre of your chest. This is very similar to the push shown on page 32, only here the left foot is forward.

3 As with all the pushes, make sure you don't get tempted to lean!

17 Turn and cross hands

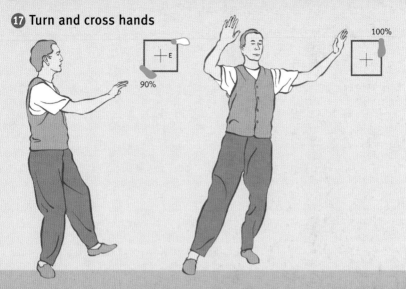

90%

+E

100%

BREATHE IN

1 Transferring most of your weight once again into the rear leg, relax your hands and lift your left toes, keeping your heel on the ground. Your hands should look rather like you are warming them in front of a fire.

2 Prepare to pivot on your left heel to turn your waist towards the south; most of your weight remains in the right foot, with your gaze directed inwards.

3 Keep those shoulders relaxed!

BREATHE OUT

1 Having turned your left foot to point as near south as you can, bring the weight back into your left side and begin to draw your right foot back, with the toes pointing south and making only the lightest of contact with the ground.

2 Meanwhile, as you turn your body towards the south, begin to separate out your hands, in what will shortly become two halves of a great circle which you will 'draw' in the air.

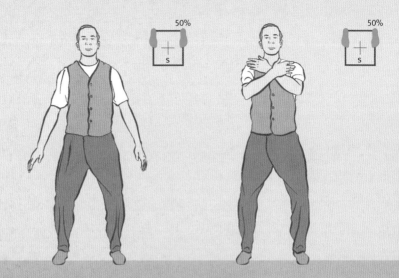

OUT-BREATH FINISHES

1 The turn concludes with the hands having descended in two sweeping arcs to complete a circle at the level of the hips.

2 Your feet should now be alongside each other in a parallel, shoulder-width stance. Just as you're finishing the out-breath, turn your palms to face slightly inwards, with your elbows well-spaced away from your sides, as though embracing a great sphere.

3 Let your weight sink down.

BREATHE IN

1 With your feet now parallel and the toes pointing south, lift your hands up through the centre of the body to cross (left wrist on top of right) at about chin height. In other words, the left forearm is closer to you than the right, as the wrists cross.

2 Keep your shoulders relaxed as you raise your arms, and don't tighten your knees. The whole of your body should remain straight, perfectly aligned and relaxed.

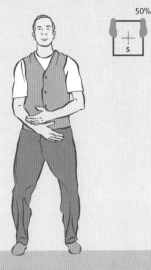

50%

S

BREATHE OUT

1 Lower both hands down through your centre and let your weight sink down. The feeling here is of sealing in the energies, and it is possible to finish your tai ji session at this point, this traditionally being the closing movement of the 'first part' of the form. Here, however, we are going to prepare for the next movements.

2 Bring a good percentage of your weight into the left side, with the back of your left hand trailing along your right forearm as you lower your hands.

finding the
diagonal

Here, we step for the first time on to the diagonal axis. Movements of this kind present a fresh challenge, helping us to develop our own sense of orientation. We are now compelled to work in relation to our own centre, without reference to our surroundings; the walls of the room, for example, are no longer of use in lining things up. This enhanced self-awareness is an important stage in the tai ji journey.

18 Carry the tiger to the mountain

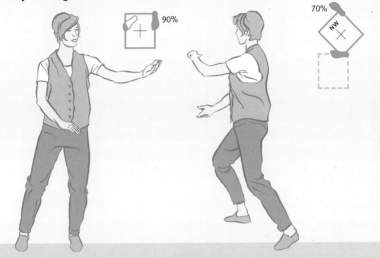

BREATHE IN

1 From turn and cross hands at the end of the previous section, uncross your hands to your left, raise your right heel and transfer your weight into your left side.

2 With your hips and shoulders facing south-east, raise your left palm to about chest height. Prepare to step around to the north-west by drawing your right toes in a little closer towards your left heel. This is a big step coming up, so make sure you feel properly balanced in your left side before commiting to the turn.

BREATHE OUT

1 Rotate your waist clockwise, and step around to set your right foot down, heel first, pointing north-west. As you go, 'brush' your right thigh with your right palm, turning it face up as your right knee bends and the weight settles in your right side.

2 At the same time, bring your left hand across, palm facing down now, to form a ball at your right side, with your right hand underneath.

3 As soon as your weight settles, adjust your back foot to a comfortable position.

⑲ Diagonal rollback and press

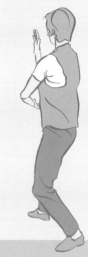

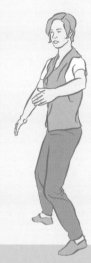

BREATHE IN

1 With your head, hips and shoulders all facing north-west, sit back into the rear leg and move your arms, raising the right and dropping the left by 'sliding' it along the right forearm to cup the right elbow.

2 This is the 'rollback' position, exactly the same as on page 30, only this time it's done towards the 'mountain', with the waist turning slightly to the right.

3 Don't lock the front knee as you sit back.

IN-BREATH FINISHES

1 Turn your waist anticlockwise and circle your left hand back, while folding your right forearm down and across your centre. Newcomers to tai ji often perceive this movement as complex and difficult to learn; just relax and let your arms find their places naturally, as your waist turns and your knees bend.

2 There should now be a little more weight in your back leg than in the previous stance.

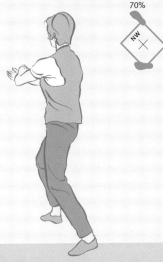

70%

NW

BREATHE OUT

1 Rotate and turn your palms to face each other, then bend your right knee, turning your waist back towards the north-west.

2 As you do this, allow your left palm to approach your right until the heels of the palms make contact very lightly in front of your chest.

3 Most of the hand energy is now concentrated in your left hand, to mirror the substantial right leg. Your hips and shoulders should now be facing north-west again.

20 Diagonal push

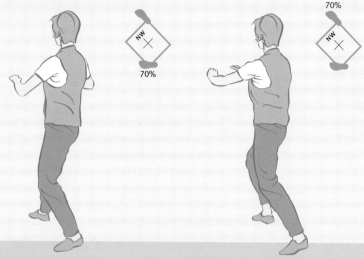

BREATHE IN

1 As before, with hips and shoulders facing north-west, separate your hands and then sit back once more into the rear leg.

2 It's worth noting here (and, in fact, this applies every time you do this movement) that as you separate your hands from the press, try to do so by trailing your right thumb across your left palm. This ensures a rolling and 'sliding-apart' appearance to the hands that is particularly smooth and pleasing.

BREATHE OUT

1 Slowly rotate your palms to face ahead, without creating a sharp angle at the wrist joint, and then, shifting your weight forward once again, push towards the north-west at about chest height.

2 Make sure your hands are relatively central; your thumbs should be about 25 cm (10 in) apart at the most, although this will depend on your overall size. You might like to cultivate a slight 'lifting' movement to the push, with your hands rising a little as they go forward.

21 Diagonal single whip

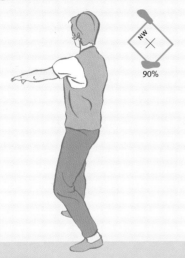
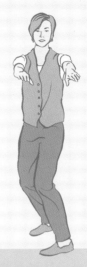

90%

90%

BREATHE IN

1 From your north-west-facing position, sit back into the rear leg and allow your arms to straighten, your palms facing downwards.

2 This time, the single whip is a real test of your spatial co-ordination by going from north-west to finish facing south-east. In every other respect, however, it is exactly the same movement as shown on pages 33–35. (NOTE: you can also find this sequence illustrated with the rest of the chorus, beginning on page 91.)

BREATHE OUT

1 With your weight mostly in the left side, pivot very slowly on your right heel to turn your waist anticlockwise, allowing your arms to follow your centre as your waist turns and your feet become slightly pigeon-toed.

2 Remember to let your waist turn freely about its axis (the spine), and to shift your weight clearly back and forth between your left and right legs, as the turning takes place.

3 Even though your arms are relatively straight, don't lock your elbows at any time.

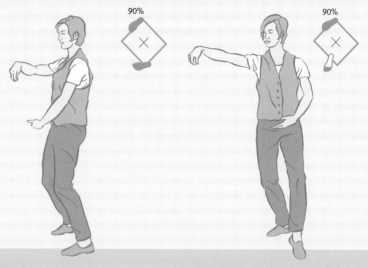

BREATHE IN

1 Now rotate your waist clockwise, while drawing the right hand back horizontally in front of your right shoulder to form the crane's beak – the wrist loose, and fingers pointing downwards, with the index finger and thumb lightly touching, like holding a pinch of salt.

2 Your left hand, meanwhile, swoops down, palm facing upwards, to settle near your right hip. Think of this movement rather like a 'scooping-up' motion, as though you were scooping up sand.

BREATHE OUT

1 With most of your weight now in the right side, pivot on your left toes by raising your left heel.

2 Turn your waist anticlockwise once more, as you straighten your right arm to project your crane's beak towards the west, keeping your gaze directed roughly in the region of your right hand as it goes.

3 Make sure you keep your elbow soft and relaxed. The arm may appear to be nearly straight, but it's not – not quite. Always keep a little in reserve.

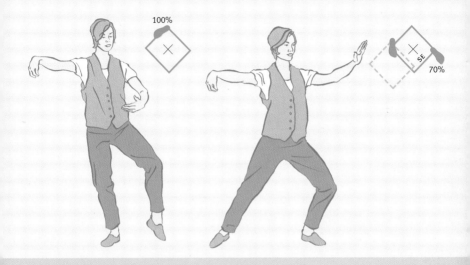

BREATHE IN

1 For the final stage, empty all the weight from your left side and prepare to step around to the south-east by drawing your left toes in a little towards your right heel.

2 At the same time, raise your left hand, palm facing in. It's useful to continue with the sand metaphor here. Having scooped it up with your left hand, now allow it to trickle from your fingers as you turn and lift the palm.

3 Keep your gaze directed towards your left palm as it rises.

BREATHE OUT

1 Now rotate your waist, step around to the south-east with your left heel, and bend your knee.

2 As soon as the weight returns to your left side, adjust the back foot to a comfortable position by pivoting on your right heel to get your hips and shoulders facing south-east.

3 Rotate your left hand to point outwards, as if towards the distant horizon, while your right arm, still extended, with crane's beak intact, remains slightly behind you, a focus of energy. Don't let your arm go weak.

22 Fist under elbow

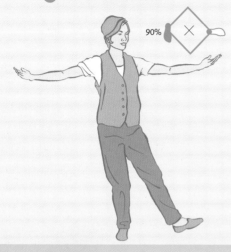

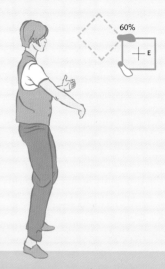

BREATHE IN

1 Now we come to another 'three-step' movement. Again, it helps to count the steps as you go. Shift the weight from your left foot and sit back into your rear leg. Let go of the crane's beak, relax your elbows and open your hands, palms up, one at a time (first the right, and then the left).

2 Next, pivot on your left heel to point the toes due east and then set your foot down flat on the ground, bending your left knee to bring the weight forward once again. That's step number one.

IN-BREATH FINISHES

1 Draw up your right foot and place it alongside the left, with the toes pointing out (step number two).

2 Bring your weight forward into your right side, allowing your waist to turn naturally to get your hips and shoulders facing east just as your in-breath is finishing.

3 Meanwhile, drop your arms around and down, slightly to your left, with your palms still open, your left hand slightly higher than your right.

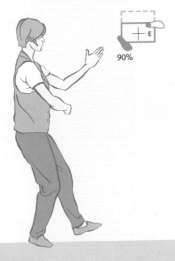

90%

BREATHE OUT

1 With your weight now in your right side, slide your left foot forward into a narrow heel stance to the east (step number three).

2 At the same time, drop your right arm a little lower and project your left hand and forearm forward and across, to point the fingers due east at chin height. The left hand should be flat, while the right hand forms a loose fist (almost as if you were holding an egg), which comes to rest just inside, to the south of the left elbow.

stepping back and stepping sideways

Some radical changes in the character of stepping occur in this section. The focus here is on the rear and the sides of the body, and on motion in these directions. Both these developments engender a further increase in our powers of co-ordination and spatial awareness, and feature sequences of wonderfully rhythmic, flowing movement.

23 Repulse monkey (right side)

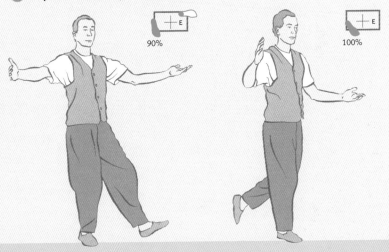

90%

100%

BREATHE IN

1 This movement is repeated three times in succession, on alternate sides. Still in the narrow heel stance from the end of the previous section, let go of the fist in your right hand and turn up your left palm. You can think of this as offering the monkey some food, tempting him to come down from the trees.

2 Turn your waist clockwise and circle your right palm back behind you, watching your hand out of the corner of your eye. Meanwhile, sink your weight into your right side.

BREATHE OUT

1 Having raised your left foot from the ground by sinking into your right side at the end of the in-breath, now step back behind with your left foot, making contact with the toes first.

2 As you step back, begin to lower your left hand to your side by bringing your elbow down and drawing it back.

3 Begin to move your right arm around to the front, in preparation for the push in the next step.

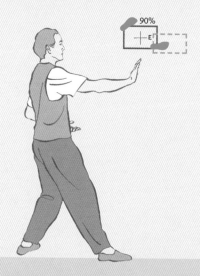

OUT-BREATH FINISHES

1 Now shift all of your weight back
   into your left foot, and push out
   towards the east with your right
   palm. You can think of this as
   pushing the monkey's nose, just as
   he comes to get the food that you
   were holding in your left hand.

2 At the end of the movement, as you
   push forward, adjust the front foot
   to turn the toes east. That is the
   end of the first repulse monkey.

24 Repulse monkey (left side)

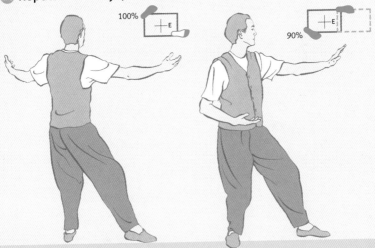

BREATHE IN

1 For the second repulse monkey we're going to repeat the previous movement, only on the other side. Begin by turning up your right palm this time, then circling back with your left hand as your waist turns anticlockwise.

2 Don't turn your waist until you have turned up your right palm. In tai ji we try to distinguish between the elements of any movement, rather than doing them all at once, as this would only dissipate the energy into too many places at the same time.

BREATHE OUT

1 Step back with the right foot, making contact with the toes first, while lowering your right hand to your side.

2 Shift all of your weight back into your right foot, and push out east with your left palm. Here, again, you are pushing the monkey's nose just as he comes to take the offering.

3 At the end of the movement, as you push forward, adjust the front foot, to turn the toes east. Keep the front foot flat on the ground once you have adjusted it. That is the end of the second repulse monkey.

25 Repulse monkey (right side)

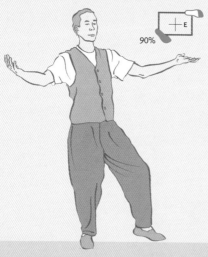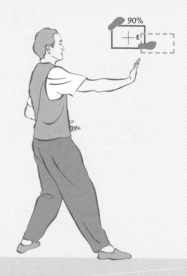

BREATHE IN

1 The third repulse monkey is much the same as the first, except that we are now coming to it from a position where the left foot is already flat on the ground, rather than from a left heel stance.

2 As before, turn up your left palm and then turn your waist to the south, and lift your right palm back behind you. The shape of the palm in all these repulse monkey movements is, once again, rather like holding a flat object, ready to hurl, but keep the arm and hand relaxed.

BREATHE OUT

1 Step back behind with your left foot, again making contact with the toes first. Simultaneously lower your left hand to your side, shift your weight back into your left foot, and push out east with your right palm.

2 At the end of the movement, adjust your front foot to turn the toes east. As your left arm descends, there should be plenty of space between your elbow and body – as if you're carrying a rolled blanket tucked under your arm (this applies to repulse monkey on the other side, too).

26 Diagonal flying

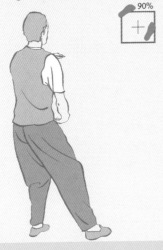

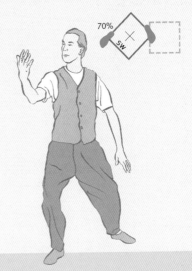

BREATHE IN

1 Staying with the image of the monkey, we are now going to pick up the monkey and help it back into the tree. Pivot on your right heel and turn your waist anticlockwise. Then, drop your right hand around near to your left hip and bring your left hand up to help form a ball towards the north-east, left hand on top, right hand underneath.

2 Then, with all your weight in your left side, draw your right toes in a little towards your left heel, in preparation for the next step.

BREATHE OUT

1 Having 'picked up' the monkey, turn your waist clockwise and step right around to put your right foot down, heel first, towards the south-west.

2 Adjust your back foot to a comfortable position and, as you turn, change your hands by raising your right arm in a great arc up towards the south-west, palm facing in, while the left hand, still retaining plenty of energy, drops back down to hip height. Your right arm should rise to the outside of your left arm — putting the monkey back in the tree.

27 Wave hands like clouds (transitional phase)

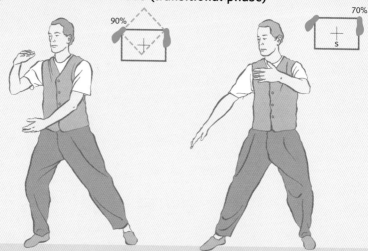

BREATHE IN

1 We now begin another sequence of movements repeated on both sides. Bring your left foot up alongside the right, at a distance of one-and-a-half shoulder widths. Make contact with your heel first, and set your foot down with the toes pointing south.

2 At the same time, swoop around with your left hand, palm down initially but changing to an inward-facing position as it goes, and bring it to settle beneath your right hand, which rotates slightly to turn palm down, to form an approximate ball.

BREATHE OUT

1 Begin to shift your weight from your right foot back across into your left side, and, as the weight changes, rotate your left palm a little to complete the ball.

2 Then change hands – that is, lower your right hand down to about hip height and raise your left to about throat height. Extend the upper arm along slightly, to make room for the lower one to rise.

3 Most of your weight has now gone into your left side, and your hips and shoulders should be facing south.

28 Wave hands like clouds (left side)

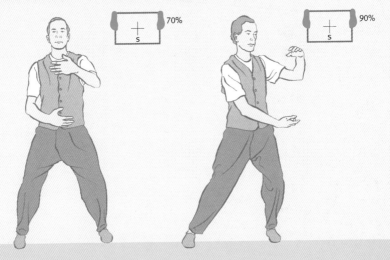

BREATHE IN

1 Tuck your right toes in to point south, parallel with your left foot, and position your hands one above the other, your left palm facing your throat, and your right palm facing your navel.

2 Your in-breath begins here, as you finish squaring up. Your hands should be a good distance away from your body – about 30 cm (12 in), depending on your own proportions and height. Keep the knees apart, 'spiralled' out.

IN-BREATH FINISHES

1 Slowly turn your waist anticlockwise and, equally slowly, rotate your wrists to form a ball between your hands, left hand on top.

2 Don't go too far with the turning of the waist! Never turn to such an extent that you introduce tension. Your knees shouldn't cave in towards each other with the turn, your waist shouldn't feel tight, and your bottom shouldn't stick out. Complete the in-breath with this turn.

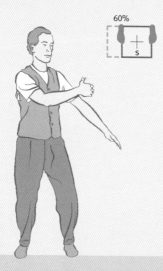

60%

BREATHE OUT

1 With most of your weight now settled
   in your left side, step inwards with
   your right foot, making it shoulder
   width from your left foot and parallel,
   toes pointing south.

2 Then, as the weight settles slightly
   more in your right side, change your
   hands by lowering the left hand and
   raising the right. Extend the upper
   arm slightly along (in this case to the
   east), to make space for the lower
   arm to rise to the inside of it.

29 Wave hands like clouds (right side)

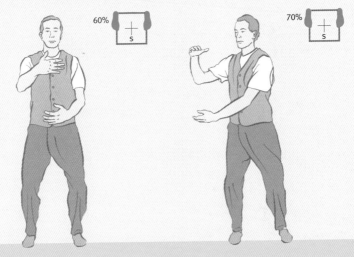

BREATHE IN

1 You are now going to repeat what you have just learned, but on the other side. Begin by turning your waist back to your south-facing position, continuing to shift your weight into your right leg as you go. This time, the right palm is positioned facing the throat, with the left palm below, facing the navel.

2 Don't linger in this position; treat it as part of the wider turn to the right, which comes next.

IN-BREATH FINISHES

1 Turning your waist clockwise, form another ball with your hands, right hand on top.

2 Don't exaggerate the ball shape; remember that in tai ji, 'holding a ball' means that an energy connection should exist between the palms. As long as you have that feeling – if only on an imaginative level at first – it's enough. You don't need to spell it out by creating a precise ball shape.

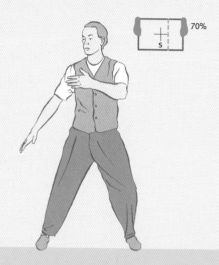

70%

S

BREATHE OUT

1 With most of your weight now in your right side, step further along towards the east with your left foot, toes still pointing south, so that there is at least one-and-a-half shoulder widths between your feet.

2 As the weight settles in your left side, change hands by lowering the right and raising the left. Again, extend the upper arm slightly along (here, to the west), to make space for the lower arm to rise to the inside of it.

③⓪ Wave hands like clouds (left side)

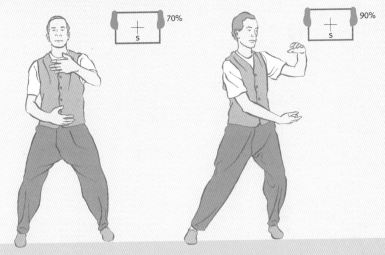

70%

90%

BREATHE IN

1 Turn back to your south-facing position – keeping your feet in the same place – with your left palm facing your throat and your right palm facing your navel.

2 It's tempting to ignore this 'squaring up' stage, and simply go straight round, turning from one side to the other. Always return to this south-facing position first, however, to get your bearings before continuing round to the side.

IN-BREATH FINISHES

1 Turn your waist anticlockwise and form a ball with your hands, left hand on top, palm down. Always rotate your wrists slowly as you form the ball, keeping your hands relaxed throughout. Be precise about this.

2 As part of the learning process, it is sometimes necessary to adopt a methodical approach at first. Be patient, concentrate, and you will soon 'free up' more during this movement.

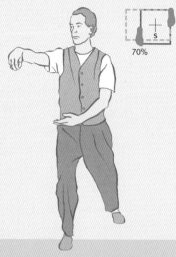

70%

BREATHE OUT

1 This time, step forward a half-pace
with your right foot, heel first, and
shift your weight forward by bending
your knee. Move your foot in as you
step, so that your feet are shoulder-
width apart.

2 Then, as your hands change, raise
your right hand in the form of a
crane's beak and turn your left palm
upwards, following round to settle
beneath, near your right hip. Your
waist can turn a little clockwise as
you go.

31 Single whip

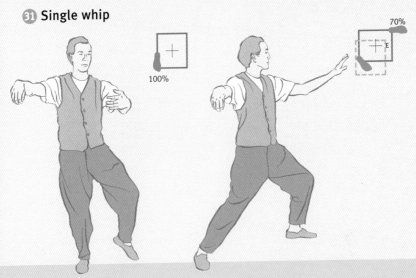

100%

70%

E

BREATHE IN

1 The final stages of the single whip conclude this section. Prepare by emptying the weight from your left foot and drawing your left toes in a little closer to your right heel, ready to step east.

2 Continue to sink your weight into your right side as you begin to raise your left palm, changing it from an upward-facing to an inward-facing position. You may find it helpful to focus your eyes on your palm, to ensure the correct orientation of your arm.

BREATHE OUT

1 With your left foot, slowly step around good and wide to the east, heel first, and bend your knee. As soon as the weight returns to your left side, adjust the back foot to get your hips and shoulders facing east.

2 Rotate your left hand to point the fingertips outwards, the elbow rounded and soft. Don't let your hand drift out to the side – it should be in line with the left side of your chest. The energy of the crane's beak in the right hand balances the energy contained in the left leg.

downwards
and upwards

In tai ji we usually try to keep a smooth, level appearance to our movements. In this section, however, things are a little different. Here, we not only dip and rise deliberately, but we also meet with stances in which one foot leaves the ground in order to kick, all of which really gets to work on those leg muscles. The focus is on keeping the 'root' – the sense of being connected firmly to the energies of the earth.

32 Snake creeps down

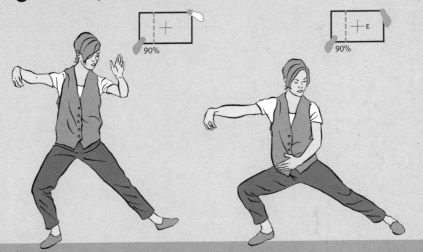

BREATHE IN

1 From the single whip position at the end of the last section, prepare for the next movement by lengthening out your stance by sliding or shuffling back with your right foot. As your foot goes back, turn it to point south-west.

2 Now bring your weight into your right leg and draw your left hand back a little towards your chest, to face roughly south-west. Keep the crane's beak intact in your right hand.

IN-BREATH FINISHES

1 Now sit back into your right leg, lowering your body into a kind of squatting position while turning a little on your left heel to point the toes of the left foot inwards, roughly south-east.

2 At the same time, continue to draw your left hand back towards your chest, flattened and blade-like, the palm now facing inwards.

3 Keep squatting as low as you can without discomfort. Try to keep your body upright – don't lean forward just to get down a few inches lower.

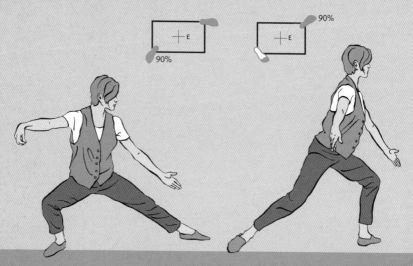

BREATHE OUT

1 Still squatting down, allow your left hand to continue on its circular sweep downwards and forwards, close to the ground, the fingers leading and the palm facing south.

2 As you move your hand past your foot, straighten your foot to point east once again. Note that there is still a slight bend to the left knee, even though the leg itself is almost straight.

3 Above all, relax! Never view your tai ji as some kind of stretching exercise; that can be done in the warm-up.

OUT-BREATH FINISHES

1 Raise your body a little and bring your weight forward, letting go of the crane's beak. This releases the weight from your right foot, enabling you to turn it inwards again, pointing towards the south-east.

2 As soon as this is accomplished, shift your weight backwards and turn your left toes out by pivoting on your heel, in readiness for the next stance.

3 Bring your weight forward once more over your left foot. As you do this, your right heel will come up to leave only the toes touching the ground.

33 Golden pheasant stands on left leg

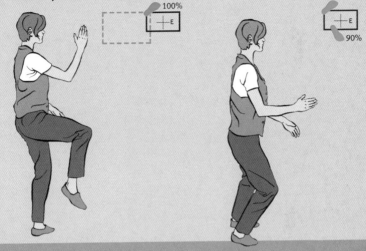

BREATHE IN

1 Begin by making sure your left knee is over your left foot, then come forward and up, raising your right knee as far as is comfortable while almost simultaneously bringing up your right forearm too, so that your elbow settles above your right knee.

2 The forearm, elbow, knee and shin should all be roughly aligned when seen from the front, and not sticking out to the side. Your right palm should be facing north, while your left hand is relaxed by your side, palm facing down.

BREATHE OUT

1 Slowly lower your right arm and leg, making sure that your right foot touches the ground alongside the left, about shoulder-width apart and with the toes pointing outwards, roughly south-east.

2 Allow your weight to settle in your right side and relax your right hand, with the fingers pointing slightly inwards and palm now facing down.

3 Sink well into your right foot in preparation for raising your left leg in the next step, to repeat the movement on the other side.

34 Golden pheasant stands on right leg

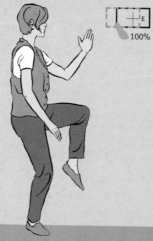

35 Pat the horse on the right

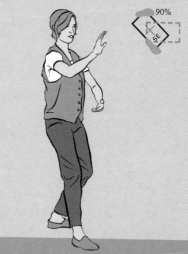

BREATHE IN

1 Once your weight is settled in your right side, slowly raise your left knee to a comfortable height along with your left arm. If your balance is poor, keep the tips of your toes on the ground; it's important to feel relaxed, and to keep the back straight.

2 Avoid creasing up or leaning over as you rise into position. If you suspect that this is happening, and your stomach feels all tense, then simply lower your knee.

3 Your right hand should be relaxed by your side, palm facing down.

BREATHE OUT

1 With your next out-breath, lower your left arm and set your left foot down slightly to the rear, making contact with the toes first.

2 As the weight settles back into your left leg, slide your right palm forward, as if resting on the flank of a horse. Meanwhile, rotate your left hand to turn palm-up, as if holding an apple for the horse to eat.

3 Keep your right hand relaxed, but note that as your weight goes into the rear leg your right palm flattens out and becomes more energized.

36 Separate hands and kick with right toes

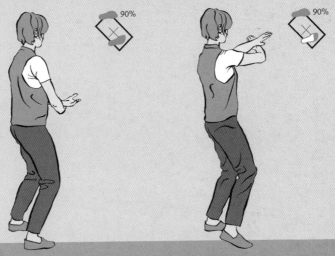

BREATHE IN

1 Turn in your right foot by pivoting on the heel to go slightly pigeon-toed.

2 At the same time, drop your right arm and cross your wrists, left wrist over right at waist level. In the process, your left hand will want to execute a little clockwise circular movement to drop down onto your right wrist, just as the right arm descends.

3 The hands should be fairly flat and blade-like, but not tense.

IN-BREATH FINISHES

1 Now raise your crossed hands to about chin-height. As your arms rise in preparation for the next phase, roll your wrists over so that the palms change from their inward-facing position to face outwards, north-east.

2 Begin to turn your right foot back towards the south-east by pivoting on the toes, which automatically lifts the knee and prepares you for the forthcoming kick.

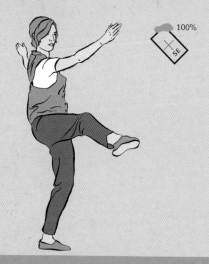

100%

BREATHE OUT

1 Continue to pivot on your right toes
   and then raise your knee as you
   separate your hands to 'draw' a
   large arc in the air: your right hand
   goes forward and your left hand
   goes back behind.

2 Then, bringing up your shin, kick
   very slowly to the south-east with
   your right foot. In this case, if you
   were actually kicking something,
   it would be the toes that make
   contact – hence the name 'kick
   with toes'.

37 Pat the horse on the left

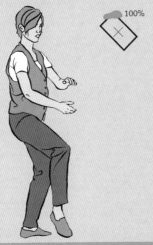

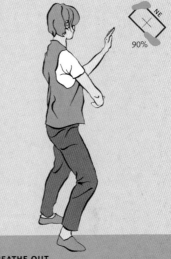

BREATHE IN

1 Still keeping your knee up, drop the shin and lower your arms inwards just a little, in preparation to step down in a moment into another pat horse (this time, on the other side, and with your weight in the front, rather than the rear, leg).

2 You may find it helpful to remember it like this: the first time you meet the horse you are cautious, so you keep back, but here, the second time around, you're more confident, so your weight goes forward.

BREATHE OUT

1 Place your right foot down just a little ahead of your left, and with the toes pointing out to the south-east.

2 Bringing your weight forward, place your left palm out to the north-east, to rest on the horse's flank, while turning your right palm up (to 'feed' the horse the apple). Again, your arms move into position across your body, the left hand sweeping over from the centre towards the north, while the right hand pulls back from the north towards the centre.

38 Separate hands and kick with left toes

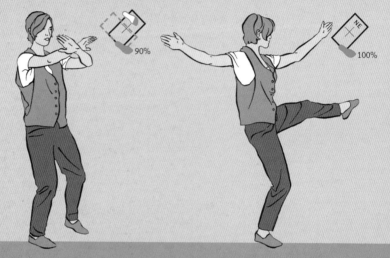

BREATHE IN

1 Step up a little with your left foot to bring it almost level with your right, and pivot on the heel to go slightly pigeon-toed.

2 At the same time, drop your left arm and cross your hands, right wrist over left, palms facing in at the level of your waist. This time, your right hand has to execute a little anticlockwise circular movement to drop down onto your left wrist.

3 Lift your hands to about chin height, rotating your wrists outwards as you go, so the palms face south-east.

BREATHE OUT

1 Pivot on your left toes and lift your knee, as you separate your hands once more to 'draw' a large arc in the air: your left hand goes forward, and your right hand goes back behind.

2 Now kick: lift the rest of your left leg and project your foot out to the north-east. Don't forget that this is another toe kick, so there is a stretch along the front aspect of the leg and foot.

3 Direct your gaze outwards – don't look down – and try to keep your hands flat and blade-like.

39 Turn and kick with heel

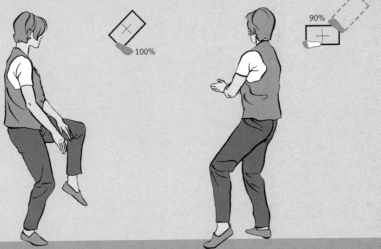

100%

90%

BREATHE IN

1 This movement involves a turn on the right heel (advanced practitioners may perform this without placing the left foot down at all). Drop your shin, keeping your knee up, and lower your arms slowly, the left arm coming down vertically across your centre, and the right arm coming to settle just to the outside of your right hip.

2 You are about to turn, to face your hips and shoulders west; as you go, let your right wrist cross over the left. This should happen naturally with the momentum of the turn.

IN-BREATH FINISHES

1 Rotate your waist anticlockwise so that you can place your left foot down behind, toes first.

2 Shifting your weight momentarily into your left foot, pivot on your right heel to get your toes pointing north-west, and then return your weight to your right foot as you raise your left knee again.

3 Your hands should have crossed by now, right wrist over left, and you can now roll them up to your chin, as before.

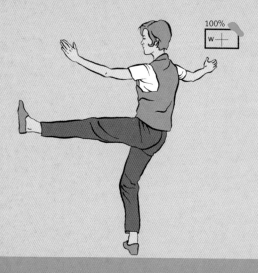

100%

BREATHE OUT

1 With your knee raised, and your hips and shoulders facing west, lift your shin and project your left foot forwards to kick. If you were making contact with anything, it would be the sole or heel of the left foot that would do so. This is a totally different feel to the previous kicks: here, there is a stretch along the back of the leg.

2 At the same time, separate out your hands in a graceful arc, the left hand going forward and the right going back.

40 Brush left knee and push

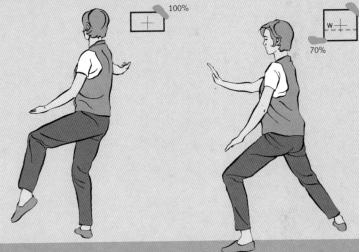

100%

W 70%

BREATHE IN

1 We now drop down into a movement already encountered earlier in the form (*see page 42*). After the kick, drop your shin and, with your knee still up, circle back a little with your right hand, palm facing up, letting your gaze follow your hand as it goes.

2 This deliberate pause, during which you take an inhalation, is a real test of your balance and ability to stay calm and steady after the impetus of the kick itself (it can be tempting to lunge forward into the next position, which is not good tai ji!).

BREATHE OUT

1 Set your left foot down good and wide, heel first, and brush your left knee with the palm of your left hand (remember the distance!).

2 Bend your knee to bring your weight forward as you push your right palm past your right ear and then onward to the west. Make sure your palm finishes centrally, not out to the side, and at about chest height.

3 Relax your left hand after the brush-knee part of this movement, so that your energy can focus itself into your right palm.

❹ Brush right knee and push

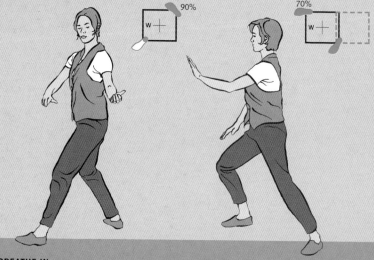

BREATHE IN

1 We are now going to repeat this sequence on the other side. Begin by establishing the yin phase, sitting back and turning out your left toes.

2 Drop your right arm to the centre while circling the left palm back behind your shoulder, palm up, letting your gaze follow your hand as it goes.

3 Try to establish an energy connection between your hands as you rotate your waist – anticlockwise – to accommodate the backward journey of your left hand. Take your time.

BREATHE OUT

1 With your weight settled in your left side, step out west with your right foot, heel first, and bend your knee to bring your weight forward.

2 As you step, brush your right knee with your right palm (keeping that distance!), your hand travelling from left to right in a sweeping motion. Then push out with your left palm towards the west.

3 Relax your right hand after the brush-knee, so that your energy can focus itself into your left palm. Your hips and shoulders should be facing west.

42 Brush left knee and punch low

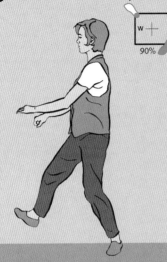
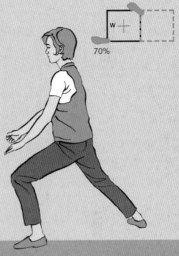

BREATHE IN

1 Shift your weight into your back leg to enable you to pivot on your front heel and turn out the toes.

2 At the same time, circle your left hand down while forming a fist with your right hand, knuckles up, by your right hip.

3 When we encountered the preparation for the punch back on page 46, the knuckles of the hand initially faced downwards. Here, they face upwards, due to the low angle of the punch. It feels more comfortable this way.

BREATHE OUT

1 Now put the whole of your right foot down and step out west with your left foot, heel first, and bend your knee. As you do so, brush your left palm over your left thigh.

2 Then project your fist forward and down a little, following it with your gaze, and rotating it through a quarter-turn to finish with the thumb side uppermost.

3 Try not to bend or lean forward as you punch; rather, just lengthen your stance and sink downwards instead.

rotating and turning

Here the emphasis is on rotational movements – work which involves twisting and turning, particularly beneficial for the lower organs of the abdomen, and for the reproductive and urinary systems. This is mainly found in a lengthy sequence called 'four corners', sometimes also known as 'fair lady works at shuttles', as the arm movements loosely resemble those of someone working at an old-fashioned loom. This section begins and ends with the chorus – grasp the bird's tail right through to the single whip.

43 Chorus: Grasp the bird's tail

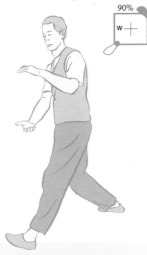

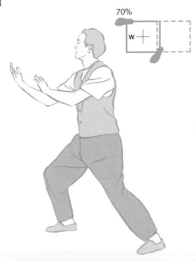

BREATHE IN

1 From your position at the end of the previous section, shift your weight back again, this time into the right side, and turn out your left toes.

2 As the weight starts to drift forward into your left leg once again, and your left foot begins to flatten onto the ground, rotate your waist anticlockwise and – from a relatively low position on your left-hand side – pick up a ball, left hand on top, right hand underneath. Keep your back upright as your waist turns.

BREATHE OUT

1 Rotate your waist back to the centre and step forward with your right foot, heel first, and bend your knee. Bring the ball with you, the ball getting smaller and smaller as you go, until you can 'grasp the bird's tail' – just like the movement you have done before (*see pages 28–29*).

2 Again, you finish up with the right arm slanting upwards and the fingers of the left hand pointing at the right palm. Remember: gently – and slowly – does it, as always.

Rollback and press

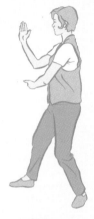 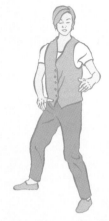 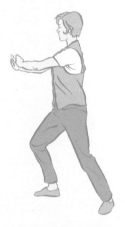

1 BREATHE IN   **2 IN-BREATH FINISHES**   **3 BREATHE OUT**

Separate hands and push

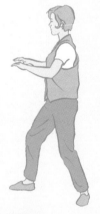 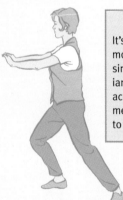

NOTE:

It's important not to treat these movements with indifference simply because they're familiar. Don't rush them! Patient acceptance of the familiar is a measure of your commitment to daily practice.

4 BREATHE IN   **5 BREATHE OUT**

Single whip

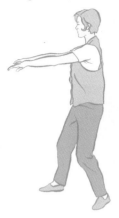

6 BREATHE IN

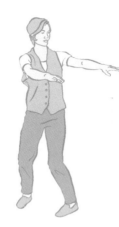

7 BREATHE OUT

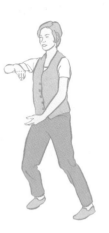

8 BREATHE IN

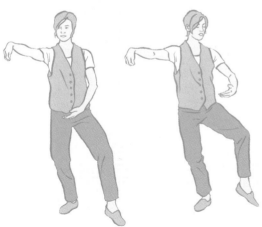

9 BREATHE OUT

10 BREATHE IN

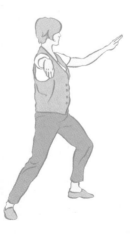

11 BREATHE OUT

44 Four corners (number one)

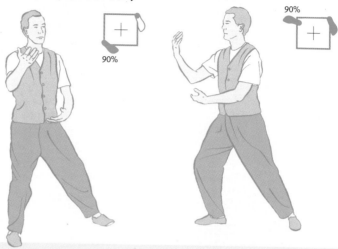

BREATHE IN

1 From the single whip, place your weight into your right side and turn on your left heel to point the toes inwards. Your waist rotates clockwise at the same time.

2 Meanwhile, let go of the crane's beak and rotate your right palm up and inwards, so that it's facing your left shoulder.

3 Then bring your right forearm back towards you, to a near-vertical position, and drop your left hand to your centre, as if to cup the right elbow at a distance.

BREATHE OUT

1 Shift the weight back across into your left side just as you begin your exhalation.

2 Then, with your waist still turning in its clockwise direction, lift your right foot from the ground and place it down again with your toes pointing roughly towards the west.

3 Finally, bring all of your weight into your right side once more by bending your right knee and sinking most of your weight into it.

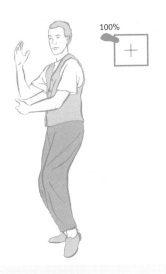

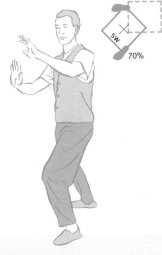

BREATHE IN

1 With all your weight in your right side, draw your left toes in a little closer to your right foot and prepare to step out towards the south-west.

2 At this stage, start to open your arms: begin to rotate your palms outwards and to raise your lower arm. Think of the left palm running up the outside of the right forearm, at a distance – not touching – and gradually let your body expand with the in-breath.

BREATHE OUT

1 Step into a wide 70/30 stance towards the south-west with your left foot, heel first, and bend your knee to bring your weight forward.

2 At the same time, raise your left hand and rotate it outwards to about head height, then rotate your right palm and push forward at about chest height. Adjust the back foot by pivoting on the heel, if necessary.

3 This concludes the first of the four corners. Your left knee and toes, hips, shoulders and palms should all be facing south-west.

45 Four corners (number two)

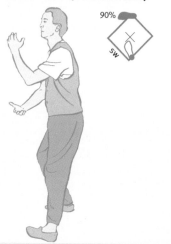

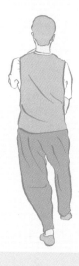

90%

SW

90%

BREATHE IN

1 Begin by emptying the weight from your left side, so that you can pivot on your left heel to point the toes as far towards the north as possible.

2 Rotate your hands inwards and draw back your arms once again – your left palm facing your right shoulder, and your right palm, having dropped to your centre, heading towards your left elbow, to adopt the same cupping configuration as before (but on the opposite side). This alternation of sides occurs on each of the corners.

BREATHE OUT

1 Transfer all your weight into your left foot as you continue to turn your waist north, and then raise your right heel to pivot on your right toes, so that the right foot is also pointing in a northerly direction. This helps to shift the body around even further on its long journey towards the south-east.

2 Remember to move from the centre of your body, as well as with the aid of the feet, and make sure you keep your shoulders relaxed and your body upright as you go.

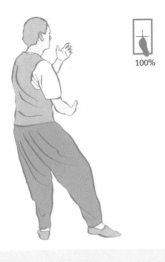

100%

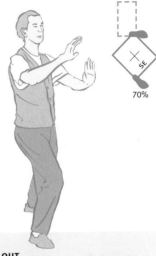

SE

70%

BREATHE IN

1 Lift your right foot entirely from the ground in preparation for stepping around to the south-east into a wide stance, and keep turning your waist clockwise.

2 Again, start to open your arms, the palms beginning to rotate outwards and the lower arm beginning to rise, all very gradually. Think of the right palm running up the outside of the left forearm at a distance.

3 Let the inhalation open your shoulders for you, and keep your back straight.

BREATHE OUT

1 Complete the turn by stepping out with your right foot into a wide stance to the south-east. Make contact with the heel first, then slowly set your foot down on the ground by bending your knee. Adjust the back foot once the weight settles in your right side.

2 Meanwhile, continue to expand your arms – right hand to head height, palm out, pushing slightly forward with your left palm at chest height.

3 That's corner number two – hips, shoulders and palms all facing south-east.

46 Four corners (number three)

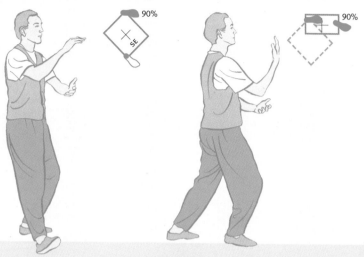

BREATHE IN

1 The approach to the third corner is more direct than for the previous two, taking us straight across to the north-east. Begin by emptying the weight from your right foot, in readiness to step.

2 Now rotate your arms slightly inwards once again – this time, rotating the right palm to face the left shoulder (the forearm moving closer to the body in a near-vertical position), and dropping the left hand to your centre, as if to cup the right elbow from a distance.

BREATHE OUT

1 With all of your weight in your left side, lift your right foot and step forwards and slightly across, to place it down flat on the ground just in front of your left foot. Try not to step in too close; there should be plenty of space between your feet.

2 Once your right foot is on the ground, bring your weight forward by bending your right knee. At this stage your head and shoulders should be facing roughly east.

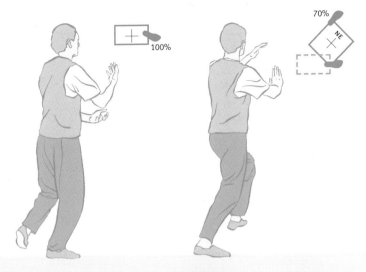

BREATHE IN

1 Sink into your right side, as you prepare to step out towards the north-east by raising your left heel.

2 At this stage, start to open out your arms again, the palms gradually beginning to rotate outwards and the lower arm beginning to rise. Think of the left palm running up the outside of the right forearm, at a distance.

3 Let your body expand with the breath. Also, start to rotate your centre, so that your hips and shoulders begin to face north-east.

BREATHE OUT

1 With all your weight settled in the right side, step out with your left heel to the north-east, and bend your knee to bring your weight forward.

2 Continue rotating and raising your left hand to head height, palm out, and then push slightly forward with your right palm at chest height. Pivot on your right heel to adjust the back foot, if necessary.

3 That concludes the third corner; left foot, hips, shoulders and palms all face north-east.

④⑦ Four corners (number four)

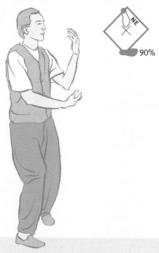

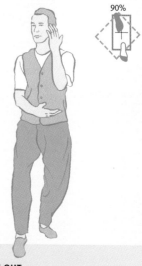

BREATHE IN

1 Start by transferring your weight back into the right side. Lower your arms and pivot on your left heel to point the toes as near south as you can, before setting your foot down.

2 Rotate your hands inwards and draw your arms back once again – the left palm facing your right shoulder, and the right palm, having dropped to your centre, near to your left elbow.

3 As you go, try to cultivate a 'rotational' feeling in the lower limbs and groin; this is most beneficial to the internal organs.

BREATHE OUT

1 Transfer all your weight into the left side, sink into your left foot and then raise your right heel to pivot on your right toes, so that your right foot is also pointing in a roughly southerly direction.

2 As you do this, rotate your waist clockwise. All this helps to shift the body round still further on its long journey to the north-west.

3 Keep your shoulders relaxed and body upright, and (except during the very early stages of learning) avoid looking down at your feet.

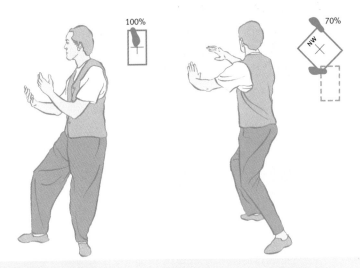

100%

70%

NW

BREATHE IN

1 Lift your right foot entirely from the ground and keep turning your waist clockwise, preparing to step around to the north-west into a wide stance.

2 At this stage, your arms start to open again, the palms beginning to rotate outwards and the lower arm beginning to rise, all very slowly and smoothly. As before, think of the right palm running up the outside of the left forearm, at a distance.

3 Let the inhalation expand your shoulders as your arms start to 'uncurl'.

BREATHE OUT

1 Still turning your waist, step out with your right foot, heel first, into a wide stance to the north-west, bending your knee to bring your weight forward. Don't forget to adjust the back foot, if necessary, once you've transferred your weight.

2 At the same time, continue to spiral out your arms – right hand to head height, palm out, while you push slightly forward with your left palm at chest height.

3 That's the final corner – hips and shoulders facing north-west.

48 Ward off left

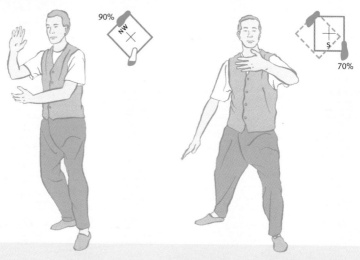

BREATHE IN

1 Rotate your palms inwards slightly and cup the right elbow. Your waist is going to rotate again, but this time in an anticlockwise direction.

2 Help this rotation along by pivoting a little, firstly on your right heel and then on your left toes, ready to step towards the south with your left foot into a wide 70/30 stance.

3 As always, check your balance before taking the final step. Meanwhile, begin to focus the hand energy largely in your right palm, ready to 'stroke' downwards.

BREATHE OUT

1 Step out to the south with your left foot, heel first, bending your knee to bring your weight forward. Continue turning your waist until your hips and shoulders face south.

2 Simultaneously, raise your left arm so that the forearm becomes horizontal, palm facing the chest, while dropping your right hand to your side. Try to sense the energy connection between the palms as they pass.

3 Remember to pivot inwards a little on your right heel, to release any tension in the back knee.

49 Chorus: Grasp the bird's tail

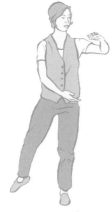 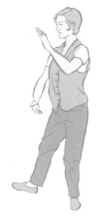 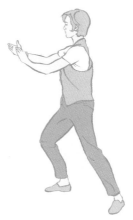

1 BREATHE IN   2 IN-BREATH FINISHES   3 BREATHE OUT

Rollback and press

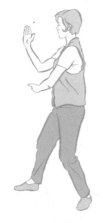 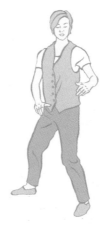 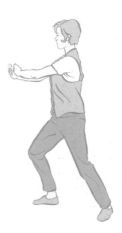

4 BREATHE IN   5 IN-BREATH FINISHES   6 BREATHE OUT

Separate hands and push

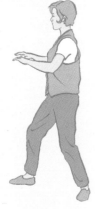

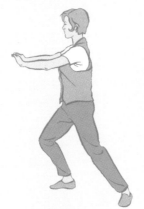

7 BREATHE IN

8 BREATHE OUT

Single whip

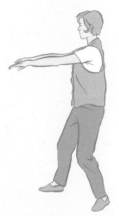

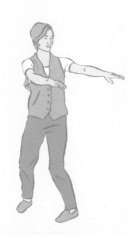

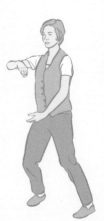

9 BREATHE IN

10 BREATHE OUT

11 BREATHE IN

Single whip continued

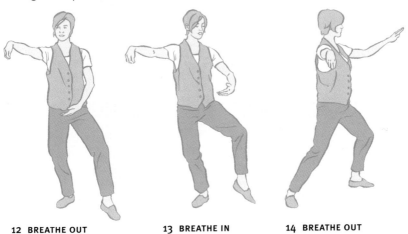

12 BREATHE OUT   13 BREATHE IN   14 BREATHE OUT

the closing sequence

Whereas the early part of the form was all about developing balance and spatial awareness, here, at the conclusion, we learn to integrate these skills with the qualities of agility and strength. The character of the movements in this closing sequence is particularly flamboyant, full of turns and extravagant sweeps of the arms – at times often quite martial in character, while at others quite breathtakingly beautiful.

50 Snake creeps down

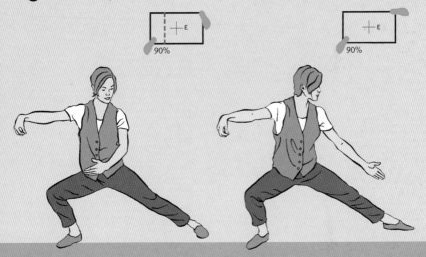

BREATHE IN

1 From the single whip at the end of the last section, we go straight into snake creeps down once again (*see also page 77*). Begin to lengthen your stance by sliding back with your right foot to point your toes south-west.

2 Sit back into your right leg and turn a little on your left heel to point your toes inwards, roughly south-east.

3 At the same time, draw your left hand back a little towards your chest, rotating the palm to face inwards.

BREATHE OUT

1 Squat down into your rear leg, your front leg remaining relatively straight, with just a slight bend to the knee, as you go.

2 Simultaneously, swoop your left hand down and then thrust it forward again, fingers first, close to the ground and with the palm facing south. Continue moving it past your left foot, which then straightens out to point east once more.

3 Keep your body as upright as possible when you sink down, but always work within your limitations.

107

51 Step forward to seven stars

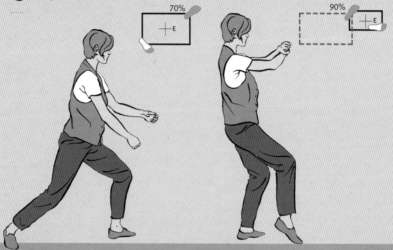

BREATHE IN

1 Raise your body a little, and bring your weight forward. This releases the weight from your right foot and enables you to turn it inwards again to a comfortable position.

2 Now shift your weight back again, and turn out your left foot by pivoting on the heel.

3 Finally, bend your left knee and bring your weight forward into the left side once more, ready to step out with the right foot. Meanwhile, move your arms in towards the centre, in preparation for the next step.

BREATHE OUT

1 With all your weight in your left side, step up with your right foot and place it down in a narrow toe stance to the east.

2 As you do this, cross your wrists, left over right, palm side of the hands facing you, having shaped your hands into two fists.

3 As you bring your body forward, roll your wrists so that the knuckle side of the hands finishes facing you. This rolling movement takes your fists up to approximately the level of your chin.

52 Step back to ride the tiger

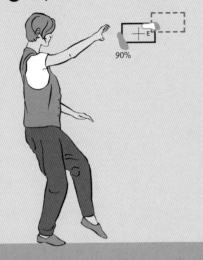

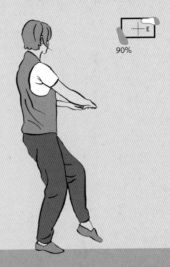

BREATHE IN

1 Uncross your wrists and open your hands. With the weight still in your left side, step back with your right foot, making contact with your toes first, then bring your weight into it.

2 Next, create a narrow toe stance on the left by raising your left foot and setting it down again properly aligned to the east.

3 At the same time, separate out your hands, the left dropping to the centre, and the right curving down and then spiralling up again to about head height, palm facing south-east.

BREATHE OUT

1 Very slowly allow your left hand to drift north, to settle above and just to the outside of your left hip.

2 Then allow your right hand, the palm outward-facing, to swoop over and down in a graceful arc, closing in once again towards the left hand.

3 Both palms should be facing downwards at the conclusion of this movement, with the fingers of the right hand pointing at the left. It's important not to raise or tense your right shoulder during this circular journey of the right hand.

53 Sweep the lotus and crescent kick

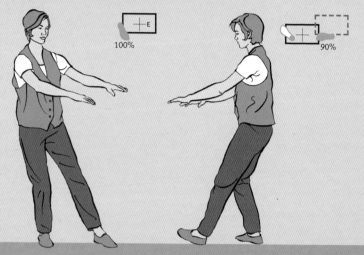

100%

90%

BREATHE IN

1 With all of your weight now in the right side, straighten out your left leg a little and raise it from the ground.

2 Using the momentum of your left leg and your arms, which are held out in front of you, sweep your body round in a clockwise direction, turning all the while on the ball of your right foot. This sweeping movement can be thought of as sweeping a lotus flower from the surface of a pool, the left foot very close to the water.

STILL BREATHING IN

1 This is the halfway stage in a 360-degree turn (the movement is illustrated in detail here, since beginners often find it quite challenging at first). At this point, you need to set your left heel down on 'dry land' to the west, and prepare for the continuation of the turn by shifting your weight into it.

2 Try not to flail out your arms in all directions as you go, but rather keep them steady and softly energized throughout.

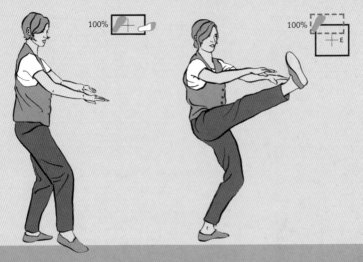

IN-BREATH FINISHES

1 Continue your turn by using the ball of your right foot and the heel of your left in combination, to bring your body round to face the east once more, in a relatively compact narrow toe stance. Your forearms continue to remain horizontal throughout the turn.

2 This turn often needs to be accomplished fairly fast, so don't be tempted to perform it slowly simply because the in-breath is demonstrated here in three stages.

BREATHE OUT

1 Allow your forearms, still horizontal, to drift a little to your right.

2 Raise your right knee and, as the shin also comes up, kick out in an arc (the 'crescent') towards the south-east. The 'kick' is the sweeping motion made by your leg as it swings round from east to south-east. If you were to make contact with anything, it would be with the outer edge of your foot.

3 As your leg sweeps to your right, your hands, still with the forearms horizontal, sweep very slightly to the left, to finish about centre.

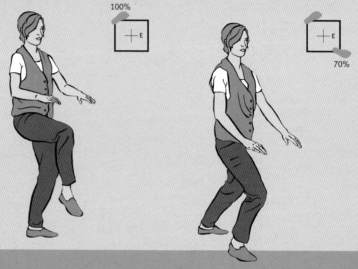

BREATHE IN

1 After the sweep and kick, it's quite enough for beginners to conclude this sequence with a dignified and steady descent back down to the ground. Always make sure you drop the shin first (keeping the knee raised), however, before you consider placing the foot down.

2 With more experience, you can try turning your waist slightly to the right to align your body and arms with your right thigh, as illustrated here. Take time to find your balance.

BREATHE OUT

1 Now set your right foot down to point south-east in a wide 70/30 stance, making contact with the heel first and bending the knee to bring your weight slowly forward.

2 Sink down and enjoy the exhalation to the full. At the same time, begin to shape your hands into loose fists level with each other at about hip height, as though you were gently clasping a thin railing. This is the 'bow' in the next movement.

3 Keep those shoulders relaxed!

54 Bend the bow and shoot the tiger

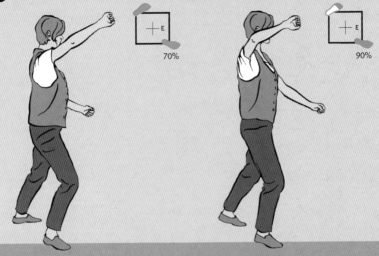

70%   90%

BREATHE IN

1 With most of your weight forward in your right side, glide the right fist up and across in a graceful sweeping curve to about head height, and with the knuckles turned inwards to face north at the top of the movement.

2 Your hand should rotate as it rises, from a palm-down position to a palm-out position at the top, meaning that your arm will have a gentle twist or spiral shape along its length. Any rotation of this kind has its origin at the elbow, but even the shoulder rotates a little as well.

BREATHE OUT

1 Allowing your waist to turn clockwise a little and, with the knuckles still turned inwards, draw your right fist back to a position close to the side of your head, while projecting your left fist forward just a moment later. This is the 'bending of the bow'.

2 The action of the left hand here is unusual, being more of a sideways, 'grazing' kind of motion – that is, outwards as well as forwards.

3 Let the back foot leave the ground a little by raising your left knee.

55 Step forward, parry and punch

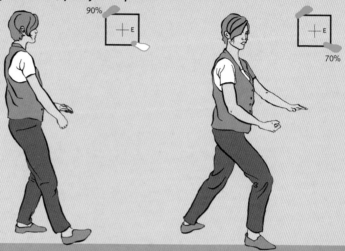

BREATHE IN

1 Allow your weight to 'rock' back into the rear leg as it makes contact with the ground again, toes first.

2 With your weight now firmly in your left side, let go of the fist in your left hand while allowing your arms to drop, both fairly central – the left hand with its open palm almost horizontal, and the right hand, still with its fist intact, hovering at about the height of the navel.

BREATHE OUT

1 The right foot is already forward, so there is no need for the first 'step' of the parry and punch sequence (remember – we counted three steps throughout the movement earlier). Instead, simply lift your right foot for a moment and then set it down again, toes pointing well out, providing a good wide base for the next stance.

2 As you do this, 'throw' your right fist around to your right side, palm side uppermost, sink into your right leg and bend your knee (equivalent to step number two of the movement).

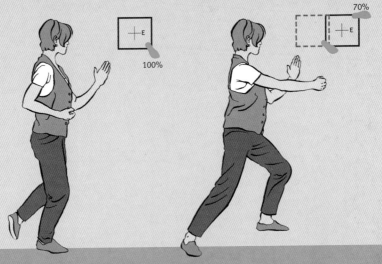

BREATHE IN

1 Prepare to step out to the east by drawing your left toes in just a little towards your right heel.

2 Allow your waist to turn slightly in a clockwise direction as you go, and draw back the fist in your right hand, knuckles still facing downwards, ready to punch.

3 At the same time, begin to raise your left forearm, ready to parry. Make sure there is plenty of space between your right elbow and your side, and that your right shoulder remains open and relaxed.

BREATHE OUT

1 Step straight ahead with your left foot, heel first (the third step). As you do this, parry with your left forearm – that is, sweep out with it towards the north from the centre.

2 Then, as your left knee bends and your weight goes forward, punch to the east very slowly. The punch should be central and roughly solar-plexus height.

3 As your fist goes forward, rotate it a quarter-turn to finish thumb side uppermost. Adjust the back heel to a comfortable position, if necessary.

56 Release arm and push

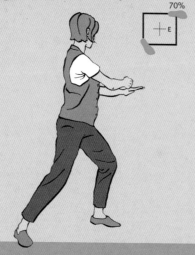

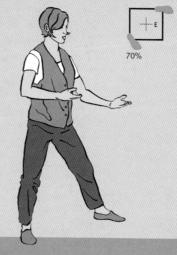

BREATHE IN

1 Begin as before (*see page 47*) by sliding the left hand under the right forearm, then turning both palms up and preparing to sit back onto the rear leg.

2 Try to cultivate a relaxed and open feeling to the hands and arms throughout, taking full advantage of the excellent rotational and loosening motions of the wrist joints that this wonderful movement provides.

IN-BREATH FINISHES

1 Now turn your waist slightly clockwise, as you bring your weight back into the right leg.

2 At the same time, draw your right hand back, with the left hand following just a moment later, coming back near to your centre, where you then rotate both wrists in preparation for the push.

3 Make sure that the front knee doesn't lock; the front leg should remain soft, with a slight bend to the knee.

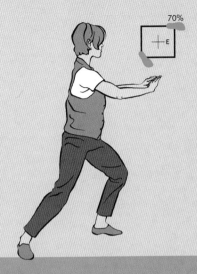

BREATHE OUT

1 Now comes the push to the east, palms facing forward. Remember that the push is generated largely through the actions of the legs, not the arms or shoulders. The shoulders should remain relaxed throughout, allowing the qi to flow into the arms and hands.

2 Make sure your weight goes forward slowly, transferring it gradually from the right leg to the left leg. Don't lean forward into the push.

57 Turn and cross hands

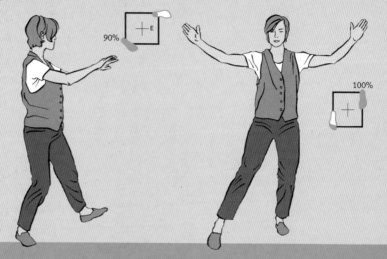

BREATHE IN

1 We meet this movement again here, to seal in the energies at the end of the entire form (it first appeared at the close of the 'first part' of the form; *see page 49*). Begin by shifting your weight to the back leg.

2 At the same time, allow your hands to relax down after the push. The shape formed by the hands is very yin-like in character, with the energy now returning inwards. In fact, the whole energy of the body can be altered from yin to yang and back again with subtle wrist movements.

BREATHE OUT

1 Pivot on your left heel to get the toes as near south-facing as you can. Then allow your weight to drift back across to the left side, enabling you to raise your right foot and draw it back, to create the parallel-feet stance with which we finish the form.

2 You can raise your toes or your heel first to draw back your foot – some people even trail the toes back along the ground. Don't lift your hands higher as you turn, but start to separate them out, as they begin to draw their great circle in the air.

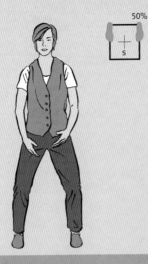

50%

OUT-BREATH FINISHES

1 Your waist having now rotated to face south, and your feet having reached their parallel position, shoulder-width apart, let your hands complete their generous, circular sweep around and down to the level of the hips.

2 The weight can now begin to settle evenly in the feet – a rare occurrence in tai ji, and one that mirrors the situation just after the start of the whole form. You are now ready for the final inhalation of the movement (*see overleaf*).

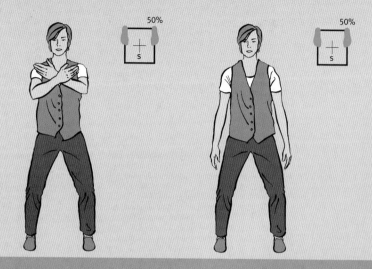

50%

S

50%

S

BREATHE IN

1 Raise your hands through the centre-line of your body, to about chin height. Here, the wrists cross, left over right – that is, with the left hand closer to your body than the right – and with the hands themselves fairly flattened in shape.

2 As always, when the hands rise up make sure your shoulders remain relaxed. Don't lose the subtle bend in the knees, either, and keep your back straight – your body perfectly aligned and balanced.

BREATHE OUT

1 Finally, to conclude the whole of the tai ji form, breathe out and slowly lower both hands down through your centre, and out to your sides.

2 Let the weight sink down as you go; bend your knees and feel the powerful contact with the earth, as the body settles into a well-rooted and yet perfectly relaxed position.

3 Keep a little space under the arms and relax the shoulders. Relax the fingers, too. That's it! Wonderful.

After the form

At the conclusion of your tai ji, always rest for a moment before moving off. Take some deep breaths and try to 'experience' how your body feels. Visualize the energy circulating freely throughout your entire body, nourishing all the vital organs and systems, and recognize that this energy is somehow a universal substance that flows through everything else around you. This is a time of repose and harmony. Enjoy it!

With practice, you will find that each time you come to the end of the form you will have returned to the same place as you began – your feet finishing on the very same piece of ground that they occupied at the start. This is an interesting feature of the short yang form, wholly practical and useful if you are working within a limited space, but also suggesting a certain cyclical character to the whole exercise.

The Chinese philosophy of life known as Taoism has always viewed the process of time as being cyclical in nature, rather than linear. In other words, things move in cycles: day follows night and returns to day again; summer follows winter and returns to summer; and so on. It is this natural law (confirmed, incidentally, by modern statistical research that has isolated literally thousands of cycles in nature and economic and political affairs) which underpins the notion of the tai ji form as a kind of journey, going forward, and taking us forward too, and yet also always returning to its source.

TIME TO REFLECT

If there is time available in your daily tai ji routine for a little reflection, then these moments immediately after the conclusion of the form can be a period of considerable illumination. For when we find ourselves at the end of the form we have, in a sense, returned from a journey. Along with the many obstacles and challenges encountered and overcome, we have each, in our own way, touched upon the great energies of nature, including several of its most powerful and mysterious creatures. The tai ji form fills our inner senses with images of tigers and cranes, populates it with snakes, horses and birds, with glimpses of strutting pheasants and mischievous monkeys. These splendid, illusive creatures, possessing such calm, dignified strength, as all wild creatures inevitably do in their natural state of health and vigour, are emulated not only outwardly in form, as we progress through the movements, but also inwardly, in spirit and instinct, every time we bring them to life.

Working in a perfectly unselfconscious, unmindful way, we should contemplate this inner vision as we go through our steps. Evoke the character of the creatures encountered on the journey, and see what they can teach us by way of being at one with the world – perfectly composed, without awkwardness, without fear of what might be, but instead living only in the ever-present 'now'. Tai ji is a journey of self-discovery – an inspiration to the spirit. That experience can never pale if it is approached in this way. No matter how often repeated, it will always have something fresh to teach us, awakening a deeper understanding each time we embark upon its mysteries.

Health benefits

When we begin life we are naturally flexible; as children, we are upright and balanced. As we grow older, however, tensions affect the body: joints become tight, the spine loses its mobility and the circulation of blood and vital fluids becomes restricted through muscular tension. Tai ji works against these trends. It is of vast benefit to our overall health, and is an excellent form of preventative medicine.

Even if the numerous statistical studies done in both China and the West are set aside, anyone who has ever done tai ji over any length of time will know how well they feel for it. So how does it work? How can the simple practice of performing a set of slow-motion movements contribute so significantly to our state of health and well-being?

Consider the nature of tai ji movement: we work slowly and calmly with the spine upright, reducing tension. With the knees slightly bent, our body weight shifts to and fro, the leg muscles working strongly to help pump blood to the heart. The arms and shoulders are in constant motion, opening and closing in graceful rotational movements, helping to stimulate the lymphatic system and improve lung capacity. We maintain the central equilibrium around the area of the *Dan Tien* – the point just beneath the navel where so much of our natural energy is gathered (*see also page 15*). The concentration and mental focus that this entails produces clarity and stability; our breathing is relaxed and constant, our metabolic rate increases, and our digestive process improves. Oxygen, blood and vital fluids circulate more easily, and the mind becomes clearer – refreshed and able to contemplate the great universal forces of ebb and flow, light and shade, and our place within nature. Being centred and happy like this in our bodies, we can apply this new-found experience and self-confidence to everything else that we do, no matter what our age or level of fitness.

An often neglected benefit of tai ji is its helpful effect on the lymphatic system. Our bodies rely on movement and exercise to encourage the circulation of lymph fluid, a substance essential for the workings of the immune system and the ability of the body to rid itself of unwanted toxins, bacteria and fungi. The non-tensile movements of tai ji are perfect in this respect, and seem to target those areas where the lymph glands are concentrated (chest, throat, armpits, groin, elbows and knees).

Tai ji is also very popular with the elderly – and it is here that the benefits are even more tangible. Studies clearly show that tai ji improves balance, and so can lower the frequency of falls (and therefore bone fractures) while also providing vital load-bearing exercise for the lower limbs, helping to maintain bone density. Regular tai ji can also help to regulate blood pressure and promotes patience and calm – useful qualities at any time of life.

TAI JI FOR HEALTH

In oriental medicine, diagnosis of illness is built around an energy-based theory rather than a viral/bacterial one, as in the West. Rather, it is the qi – the vital energy that flows through all things and is responsible for the life within us all, at every level – that is the basis of all physiological processes. A blockage or disturbance to the flow of qi, depriving the vital organs of their natural power source, is considered paramount in the process of disease. This is why it is so important to maintain its circulation.

The following pages give some examples of how tai ji movements are believed to relate to our health. Do bear in mind, however, that although some movements are considered especially helpful for particular areas, the strength of tai ji in health terms is found in its overall effect. In other words, instead of a therapy such as acupuncture, which can target specific illness, tai ji works on the immune system as a whole, and so assists the body in finding its own natural level of well-being – a state in which illness is no longer able to thrive or gain a foothold so easily. But remember: tai ji is not a cure for illness. Never view it as a substitute for medical advice.

▶ The chorus movements like 'separate hands and push' and 'grasp the bird's tail' are considered helpful for strengthening the energies of the lungs.

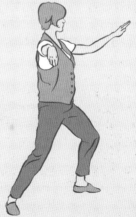

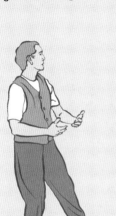

◀ Relaxed rotations of the wrist such as those found in 'release arm and push' have positive implications for the health of these joints and the numerous nerves and blood vessels that pass through them.

▶ 'Single whip', and the squatting version of this movement, 'snake creeps down', can benefit the abdominal organs by relieving any stagnation of energy or blood that can occur in these areas.

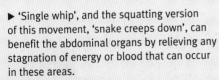

▶ The emphasis of weight distribution constantly flowing from leg to leg is very helpful in providing load-bearing exercise for the legs, and can help delay the onset of diseases such as osteoporosis in the elderly. 'Golden pheasant' is a very obvious example.

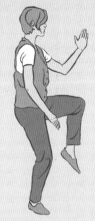

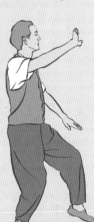

◀ 'Crane spreads its wings' is said to benefit the spine and the central nervous system via the gentle stretching and twisting it creates in the spinal column.

▶ All the heel stances and heel kicks are helpful for stimulating the circulatory system, especially the return flow of venous blood to the heart from the lower extremities.

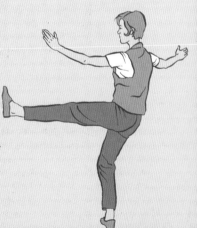

▶ The gentle turning movements of 'wave hands like clouds' are legendary for their benefits to the digestive system and to the stomach in particular, allowing the stomach to settle its energies and become calm.

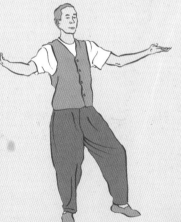

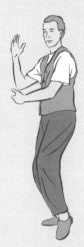

◀ The gradual twisting and rotating movements of 'four corners' help to disperse stagnation in the hips and also throughout the urinary/reproductive system.

▶ 'Repulse monkey' and other expansive movements of the shoulders assist in the circulation of lymphatic fluid around the body, essential for dealing with toxins in the body.

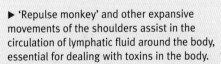

ABOUT THE AUTHOR

Robert Parry is a practitioner of oriental medicine with a special interest in traditional approaches to health and fitness, including tai ji, yoga and qi gong. He has been actively engaged in studying and writing about the health and relaxation aspects of these subjects for over twenty years, and has taught extensively at Adult Education level in the UK. Previous titles in this field include *Tai Chi for Health and Vitality*, *The Tai Chi Manual* and *Teach Yourself Tai Chi*.

Visit Robert's website at: www.orientalexercise.wanadoo.co.uk

EDDISON • SADD EDITIONS

Editorial Director *Ian Jackson*
Managing Editor *Tessa Monina*
Proofreader *Nikky Twyman*
Art Director *Elaine Partington*
Designer *Malcolm Smythe*
Production *Sarah Rooney*